DIY
Bridal Makeup
10 Steps to Flawless Wedding Day Makeup

Toni Thomas

Keisha Garrett

Published by Women in Gear, LLC

1st Edition

Copyright © 2017

Toni Thomas & Keisha Garrett

ISBN: 0692907033
ISBN-13: 978-0-692-90703-0

An application to catalog this title has been submitted to the Library of Congress.

While the authors have made every effort to provide accurate telephone numbers, website addresses, and other contact informational the time of publication, neither the publisher or the author assumes responsibility for errors or changes that occur after publication.

We teach beauty, you create beautiful.

This book is dedicated to every bride who wants to achieve a flawless look on her wedding day.
We wish you a lifetime of joy and success and the most beautiful wedding day ever.

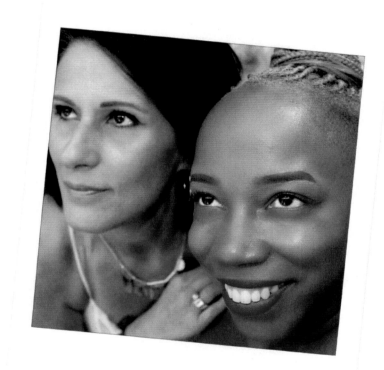

Toni & Keisha

CONTENTS

I began my career in the bridal industry twenty five years ago working as an assistant in a bridal shop; my job was to sell wedding gowns, do fittings and then alter the dresses. I was fortunate to learn how to sell in that shop and as it turns out I was pretty good at it, I was even more fortunate to get an education from the owner on how to do fittings and alterations for wedding gowns. This new skill would serve me well later in my life.

A year into my bridal shop gig we moved locations into a larger store and I became even more proficient at selling wedding gowns and developed a unique talent for making a stressed out bride-to-be feel relaxed and at ease in the crazy final days of dress fittings and final preparations. I learned I had a true talent for making others feel at ease in hectic situations that are often heightened by the situation and not the circumstances. I also traveled a bit learning the ins and outs of the retail business and what styling a bride is all about, I loved the travel and knew one day traveling for my career would be my ultimate goal.

Two years into the job I recognized that beauty comes in many forms and that every bride has a vision of how her wedding day should look, including how her bridal makeup should appear and how it should be applied, the problem seemed to be, who should apply it?

The everyday woman isn't a makeup artist and often believes she lacks the skills to do a professional makeup application on her wedding day. This I now know just isn't true, any woman with the right tools and the makeup confidence can achieve a flawless makeup application.

It became apparent to me that I could enter the beauty business seamlessly and become an entrepreneur in an industry that was beginning to be in high demand and would fit well with my artistic personality and entrepreneurial spirit. It seemed a natural transition to go in the direction of beauty and the business of beauty and I knew my decision at this point was suited to help women achieve their most beautiful self.

I entered the world of beauty first as a salon owner and then went to school to become a nail technician; this was an industry that was just taking off in the early nineties. A few years later I continued on with my education and became a licensed esthetician and certified master makeup artist, then in an unexpected turn of events I was asked to teach in the profession I had come to love and thus began my career as a beauty educator.

Twenty three years later the beauty industry has given me a clear vision of how to share my knowledge, educating those who seek to find their inner most beauty and project that beauty upon the world around them.

I am and always will be driven to share what I love with others!

-Toni Thomas

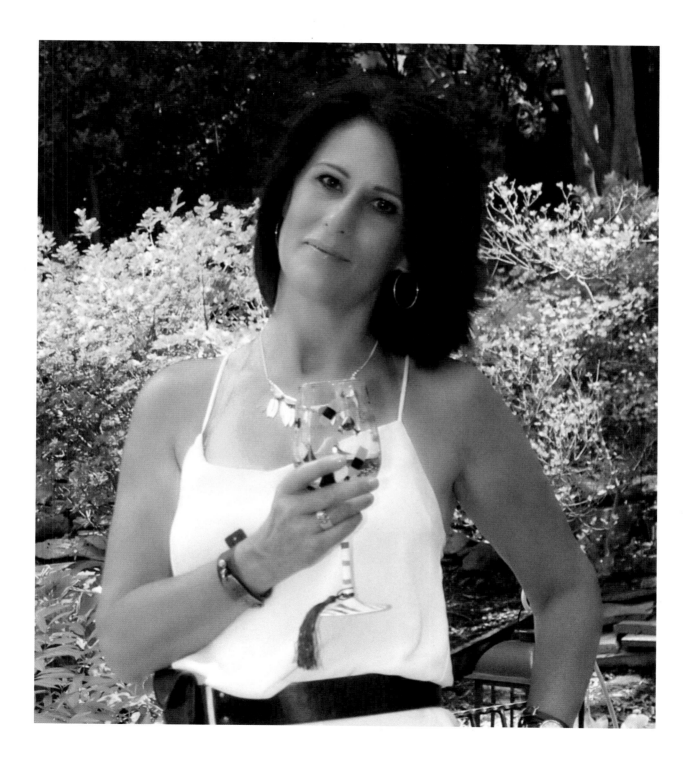

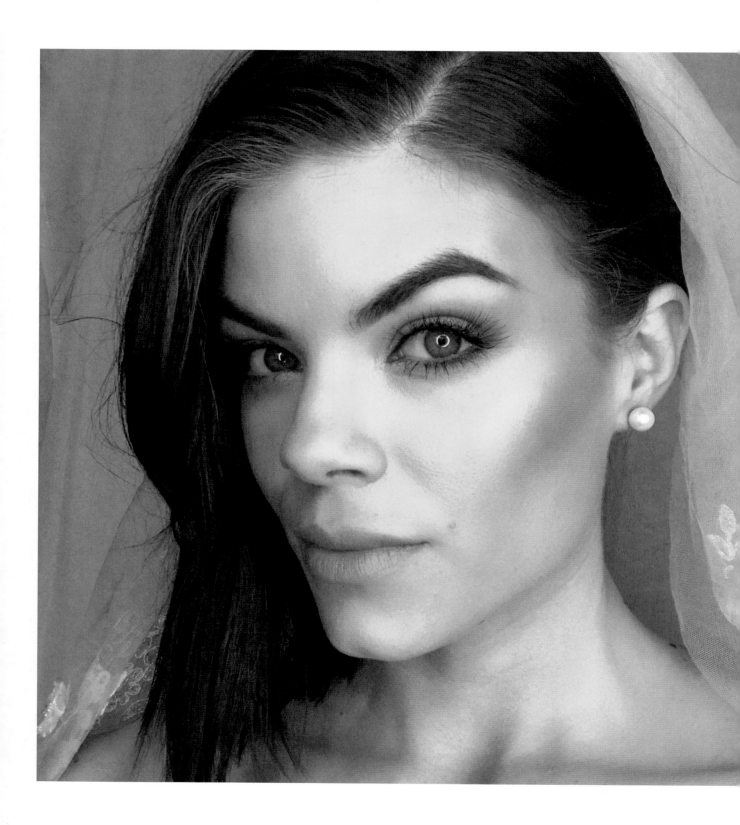

Makeup Confidence

Go confidently in your journey to enhance the beauty of you.

The wedding day has arrived, that wonderful and oh-so-stressful day that a woman spends her youth dreaming about. For most of us becoming a bride is about achieving the most beautiful and romantic look of our lives and yet it comes with high expectations and an abundance of stress. You want to look flawless and glowing as you walk down the isle to meet your beloved groom and you want every guest to have a day that they will remember forever. No wonder a bride often forgets about the wedding day makeup until the wedding has almost arrived. With so many decisions to make in the wedding planning the wedding makeup is often easily forgotten about until a few weeks before the big day, then it becomes another decision you have to make.

Do you hire a professional makeup artist to do your makeup or do you do it yourself? Will you get the results you want with a professional or is it better to rely on your daily makeup routine? As the bride you have to make the right choice for you, do you hire a professional makeup artist or do you add the makeup to your list of responsibilities? This has long been a question many brides face and often struggle over in the final few weeks of the wedding preparations. Assessing the landscape of your skills and creating a makeup plan will help you decide the best option for you.

Makeup Plan

You dream of relaxing in a chair in front of a mirror on the biggest day of your life letting someone else pamper you and make you look oh so beautiful. This is a lovely thought, hiring a makeup professional can be a great experience but it can also turn into a brides worst nightmare if things go wrong, as they often do. Wedding day pampering dreams can be shattered by a late arrival, a cancelation, or a makeup application that a bride just doesn't like, and in any one of these situations it can leave the bride and her family scrambling to deal with doing the makeup themselves. I often hear these words from past brides who decided to get a professional makeup artist or a friend to do the wedding day makeup, "I looked in the mirror and I didn't even recognize myself, I ran to the ladies room, and washed it all off then re-applied my own makeup."

It's always a bonus to hire a professional to do the wedding day bridal makeup, it's even better if that professional has done your makeup before and you know they are reliable and do a fantastic job. Unfortunately most brides hire a makeup artist they have never worked with before or they let a friend do their wedding day makeup and often they are disappointed with the results. And how do you tell your best friend you don't like the makeup application they so generously gave to you as a wedding day gift?

If you have worked with a professional makeup artist before and you are comfortable they can achieve the look you want, then by all means have your makeup done by the pro. But if that isn't the case then there are a few ways you can achieve a flawless and glowing look on your wedding day by doing your own makeup and get the professional results you are looking for.

Wedding day makeup never looked so good or was so easy to achieve when done by a bride who has learned the skills to do flawless wedding day makeup on herself.

Your desire to have a beautiful you on your wedding starts with gaining confidence in your makeup application skills and knowing what's truly important when it comes to the presentation of your bridal makeup. The key to bridal makeup success will require practicing what you learn, understanding how to apply makeup, using the right tools, and gaining the knowledge about quality makeup and which colors best suit you.

Bridal Makeup

Bridal makeup is as special as you are and no two brides are alike, each bride has a vision for her wedding day makeup look and each bride deserves to look exactly as she has dreamed of since she was a little girl.

With so many makeup application options how can you achieve the right look for you?

The great thing about makeup is there are no rules, makeup is a creative process that let's the person who is applying the makeup be as original and unique as they choose to be or as structured as is necessary, but when it comes to bridal makeup there are a few guidelines to follow.

- ☐ Perfectly matched foundation color is essential, it should be an exact match to your skin tone and look dewy once applied.

- ☐ Romantic eyes with a less is more approach will bring your face forward showcasing the eyes, and giving depth to your wedding day pictures.

- ☐ Perfectly applied blush using a two color application will give you lasting results that will carry you through the long wedding day festivities.

- ☐ Subtle contouring can give you an instant facelift and project a confident you.

- ☐ Highlighter will bring a radiant glow to your face creating a luminous look.

Makeup Balance

Bridal makeup needs to reflect not only your personality and enhance your own inner beauty but it will also need to counter balance your wedding gown. If you are wearing a white dress you will need to brighten your cheeks and lips to bring life to your face and overcome all the white reflections the dress and the wedding venue surroundings will bring. If you are wearing a beige or off white gown you will want to enhance your eyes with deeper hues to offset the cream tones of the dress and use a bronzer to give your skin a kiss of sunshine. If you are wearing bright colors that are found in some cultural weddings you will need to cool down your makeup options and enhance your eyes with charcoal eye liner that will give your eyes the pop they need to really stand out, accentuating your lashes with extra coats of mascara and or applying false lashes. Finding balance in your look will give you that pulled together polished finish exuding a confident bride who knows this is the most important day of her life.

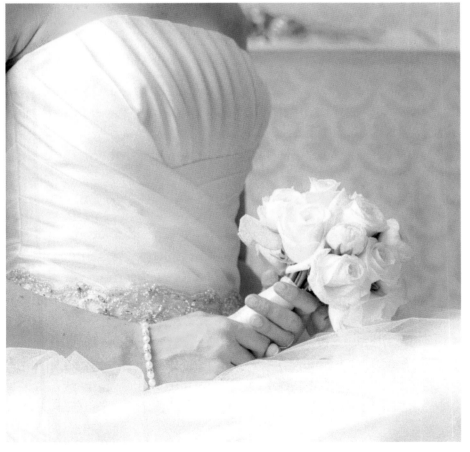

No matter what color dress you're wearing your wedding day is the day to let your dress have its moment in the limelight and your face the radiant glow it deserves.

Ethereal Beauty

On your wedding day you want to portray an ethereal beauty that sets the stage for the most romantic and memorable day of your life, so this is a day to steer clear of heavy makeup or trendy new looks that will not enhance your inner and outer beauty. Your wedding day is the day to project a healthy beautiful extension of you, this is the day to boost your own beautiful features and present your groom with a radiant bride.

Your wedding day makeup needs to be as flawless as possible and to achieve flawless you need to have makeup confidence, this means you will know how to apply your makeup so it appears as if it were applied by a professional. This means perfectly matched makeup in the right hues and tones that goes on smooth and is evenly applied over the entire face, chin, neck and chest with our blending technique that gives the appearance of airbrush makeup without using an airbrush.

An airbrush look without the use of an airbrush, can it be done?

Yes is can, and this guide is going to show you how to get that look as well as many other tips, tricks and secrets to achieving that flawless wedding day makeup application.

In the following sections you are going to learn our exclusive **10 step bridal makeup application** that will ensure you are the most beautiful you on the most special day of your life. If you follow the steps and practice each application using the rights tools and products you will have the makeup confidence to create the most beautiful you on your wedding day.

Makeup confidence starts with understanding the three key elements in makeup, even the most confident makeup artist will tell you she had to practice her skills on many faces before perfecting her techniques. She has spent countless hours practicing her techniques to achieve the proficiencies to apply flawless and well executed makeup. A makeup artists number one asset is the brushes she uses to apply makeup on her clients and to have makeup success she must use high quality makeup applied with professional grade brushes and she blends her product well to get a flawless finish. Although makeup has no rules there are a few simple techniques in bridal makeup that will need to follow to give you the results you are looking for as you build your knowledge base and gain the confidence required to have the most success in your wedding day makeup application.

3 Key Elements in Bridal Makeup

1. Practice: I can't stress enough how important it is for you to practice the skills you will learn in this guidebook. Each day you will need to practice all the steps or certain application elements that you may struggle with to give you the advantage of a flawless finish on your big day. This practice will in turn give you the makeup confidence you need for a successful application on your wedding day. By practicing everyday you will be surprised how many compliments you will receive about how beautiful and glowing you look, thus ensuring your makeup confidence even more.

2. Tools: Your tools will be an important aspect of your makeup application. And finding good quality brushes for each technique is a good investment not only in your bridal tool kit but also in all the makeup you will do for the rest of your life. Test your new brushes, do they feel good in your hand, do they put down the product the way they were designed, are they easy to maneuver in your hand, and are the bristles held firmly in the ferrule of the brush and not coming off on your face?

3. Makeup & Blending: Sounds so simple right? Apply the makeup and then blend it all in! The truth is choosing the right makeup is going to be a very important step in your makeup application success. Makeup is a multi-billion dollar industry and this means that you the consumer have many choices. Some makeup is good, some makeup is bad but most are somewhere in the middle. It doesn't really matter what makeup brand you choose, just choose a quality brand that works well with your skin, matches your skin tone, and isn't harmful to your skin. There is nothing worse than bad makeup that is also harmful to you and your skin. So take some time, get to know what works best for you and what products you like to use. Get familiar with products, go to cosmetic counters and get samples, if your friends are selling a makeup or skincare brand, ask for samples. The most common element of professional makeup artistry is blending, yes blending is everything, it adds time to the application but can be the difference in a poorly done makeup application to a spectacular makeup application. I say, "blend like your wedding photos depend on it!"

Bridal Skincare

Beauty lies in the skin and for the bride-to-be it is in the skincare regimen.

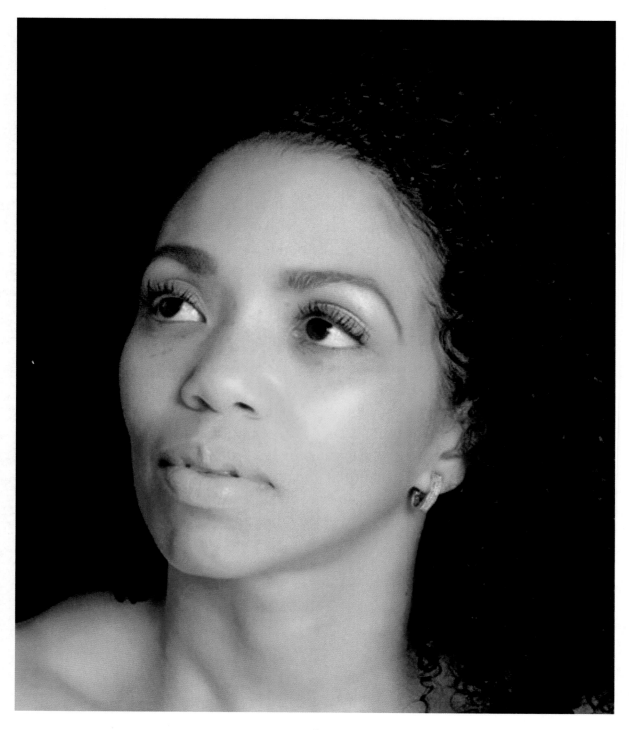

Did you know you can only feed your skin from within? Most topical beauty products and their applications do not nourish our skin, they are designed to protect and maintain our skin not to feed or repair. A balanced diet and pure water are the most precious gifts we can give our skin and a lack of water is the principal cause of daytime fatigue and under eye bags. Good skincare as well as a well balanced diet is the first step in a great wedding day makeup application and it is up to you to start your skincare routine as soon as possible and stick to it right up to the day of your wedding.

As a bride it is your responsibility to prepare your skin for the biggest day of your life. Proper skincare is important because the skin is the canvas you will lay down your makeup on, and it needs to be healthy, plump and free of skin issues. With that in mind remember the secret to healthy, beautiful, and glowing skin is drinking your daily recommend amount of water to maintain that healthy glow.

What is the recommended daily amount of water you need?

Use this simple water rule to calculate your needed water intake. Divide your body weight by 16 and the resulting number is the recommended daily amount of water you need to consume everyday. The skin is made up of 70% water and needs as much hydration as possible to keep if looking its optimal best. Studies show that 75% of the US population is dehydrated, and many Americans are functioning in a state of chronic dehydration. With this knowledge it is easy to see why many women have skin issues that give the appearance of fine lines, bags under the eyes and a less than a healthy glow we are seeking from our skin. Solving some skin issues could be as easy as drinking plenty of water and seeking the advice of a skincare professional.

Skincare Professional

Before you begin your skincare routine and at least six weeks before your wedding day we recommend seeking the advice of a skincare professional. Better yet make an appointment for a facial at your local spa or salon, get an analysis of your skin and let an expert recommend the best skincare routine based on the skin analysis you receive.

If we can only feed the body and skin from within what is the point of good skincare? Why should we use quality skincare and not just soap and water? According to Kate Tart, lead esthetician for Derma E, "applying your skin care products in the proper order ensures that your skin receives the full benefits of each product." For example, if you applied a cream-based product first followed by a serum, the cream's emolliency would prevent the serum from reaching the skin. Many moisturizers also contain water, and if you apply a moisturizer over a sunscreen, you would in effect be watering down your sunscreen and diluting its efficacy. Aside from the order of application, it's also important to consider the time it takes for your skin to absorb your products. Did You Know? Benzoyl peroxide, which is commonly found in acne-treatment regimens, has a one-to three-hour activation time, and any cream or lotion that comes in contact with it before it has completed it's work will likely inhibit the active ingredient from working properly.

Skincare is not the only thing you should consider in your skincare routine, you should also be using moisturizers and body lotions that have SPF protection. Did you know that applying an SPF sunscreen is necessary not only for long term healthy and beautiful skin but for short term as well? SPF or sun protection factor comes in various sun blocking abilities but even the highest level SPF must be re-applied every 2-3 hours to be effective. According to Web MD, an SPF 15 product blocks about 94% of UVB rays; an SPF 30 product blocks 97% of UVB rays; and an SPF 45 product blocks about 98% of rays. Sunscreens with higher SPF ratings block slightly more UVB rays, but none offers 100% protection and as we said before you should be reapplying your SPF every 2-3 hours to maintain protection.

Know that some wedding photographers discourage the application of SPF products on the day of the wedding and for any bridal or engagement photo shoots. SPF is know to cause what photographers call ghost face flash backs that make you pale and gives off a dusty white cast on photos.

The Skincare Routine

Your skincare routine is a very important element when trying to achieve a flawless makeup application on your wedding day. How your skin is functioning will have an impact on your appearance the day you walk down the isle. Skincare is a lifestyle decision and should be a part of your everyday routine. If you don't currently have a routine it is a good idea to start looking at skincare products and what you should be using.

A solid skincare routine should start at least six months before the wedding but at the very least six weeks prior to your wedding day. I recommend consulting a professional for a skincare analysis and a facial to jump start your healthy skincare routine. A skincare professional can get you started on a healthy skincare routine that will get you the right products suited for your skin and a structured regimen to get your skin functioning properly. Let the professional guide you on your skincare products and listen to their recommendations, they are the pros and have been trained to guide you to your most healthy skin. Water is essential to luminous and glowing skin but even more important is a healthy diet of fresh fruits and vegetables, plant proteins, and lean cuts of meat and fish. It is up to you to avoid foods that can cause skin irritations and outbreaks, so choose to love your skin and give it the nutrients it needs to flourish. Beauty begins with healthy skin and healthy skin begins with a balanced diet and lifestyle. It's time to become your skins BFF.

- *Eat Right*
- *Exercise regularly*
- *Sleep 8-9 hours per night*
- *Restrict sun exposure*
- *Avoid pollutants and smoke*
- *Don't over indulge in alcohol*
- *Minimize stress in your life*

These are only a few steps to take in your skincare routine. As we said before it is always a good idea to consult with an esthetician or dermatologist and get a skincare consultation before starting your skincare routine. These professionals can guide you in the right direction with the best products to use and help you get an understanding of your skin and what will be required to maintain it for it's optimal condition.

Few people have perfect skin, in fact no one is immune to skin issues and skin conditions, there are just to many factors that can affect the balance of our delicate skin. Our skin is not only affected by what we ingest into our system but even the air around us can cause skin issues. So it will be up to you to get familiar with your skin and become your skin's best friend, only then can you have your best skin ever.

Listen to what your skin is telling you, track your skins progress with a journal, and try to get a deep understanding of how your skin wants to be treated. Even sensitive and troubled skin can be transformed into a glowing canvas for you to work with as you move into your daily makeup routine.

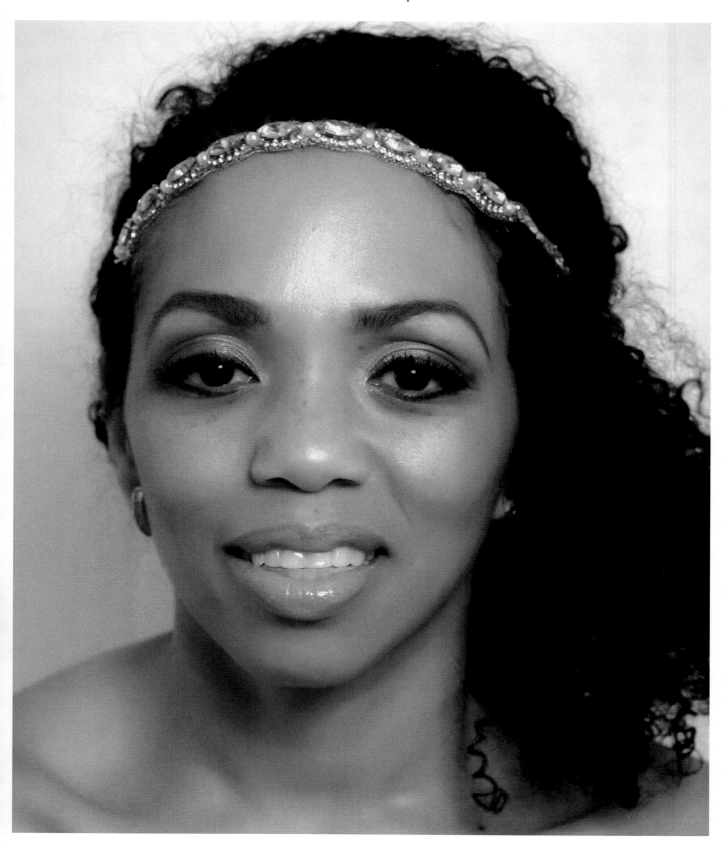

Understanding Your Skin Type

After washing your face it's?

- ☐ *Tight and a little stretched - Dry.*
- ☐ *Clean, but shiny within 20min - Oily.*
- ☐ *In good condition - Normal.*
- ☐ *Shiny in the "T" zone - Mixed.*
- ☐ *A little red and stings - Sensitive.*

When you don't use lotions your skin is?

- ☐ *Rough and scaly. - Dry.*
- ☐ *Greasy, shiny - Oily.*
- ☐ *Same as the previous day - Normal*
- ☐ *Shiny on the forehead - Mixed.*
- ☐ *Redness and scaling on cheeks or around nostrils - Sensitive.*

The skin is the largest organ in our bodies and consists of 70% water so getting familiar with your skin and your skin type is an important part of getting to know more about yourself and understanding how you can care for your skin. Understanding how your skin reacts to products, environment and even to changes in diet as well as activity is key to knowing how to care for your most precious commodity.

Therefore getting a good understanding of your skin type is one of the first steps in your skincare routine. It will be up to you to seek guidance from a skincare specialist who can guide you to the right products and who will give you a skincare roadmap to follow.

This roadmap should be well a part of your daily routine for at least six weeks leading up to your wedding day.

A Youthful Glow

The skin is our protective barrier against harmful agents such as bacteria, chemicals, ultraviolet rays, pollutants and even water absorption. It is made up of 70% water and is your greatest asset to protest and nourish. Your skin type can be easily determined and your skincare routine will be based on your skin type.

Whatever your skin type there are three basic things to remember to keep it looking youthful and healthy.

☐ *Clean it daily and always remove all make up.*

☐ *Moisturize and care for your skin with products that suit your needs.*

☐ *Protect your skin from external elements like the sun, smoke, wind, air conditioning, etc.*

A youthful glow no matter what your age can be achieved by making your skin and your skincare routine a top priority. This means planning to be committed to your skincare routine and skincare diet for up to six months prior to your wedding day. Once you have established your skincare routine and diet it will just become a part of your everyday routine.

Your skin is going to last you a lifetime and needs you to care for it as you would a new born baby, with love, tenderness and great kindness.

The saying, "love the skin you're in" is a truth most of us can't ignore.

Take the time to understand your skin type and give it the love it needs to give you that youthful and timeless glow. Your skin and your Selfies will love you for it.

Maintaining a youthful glow is easy if you take the time to love your skin from within. You must also protect it with the right products that will nurture it on the outside and keep it soft and supple and safe from harmful UV rays and pollutants.

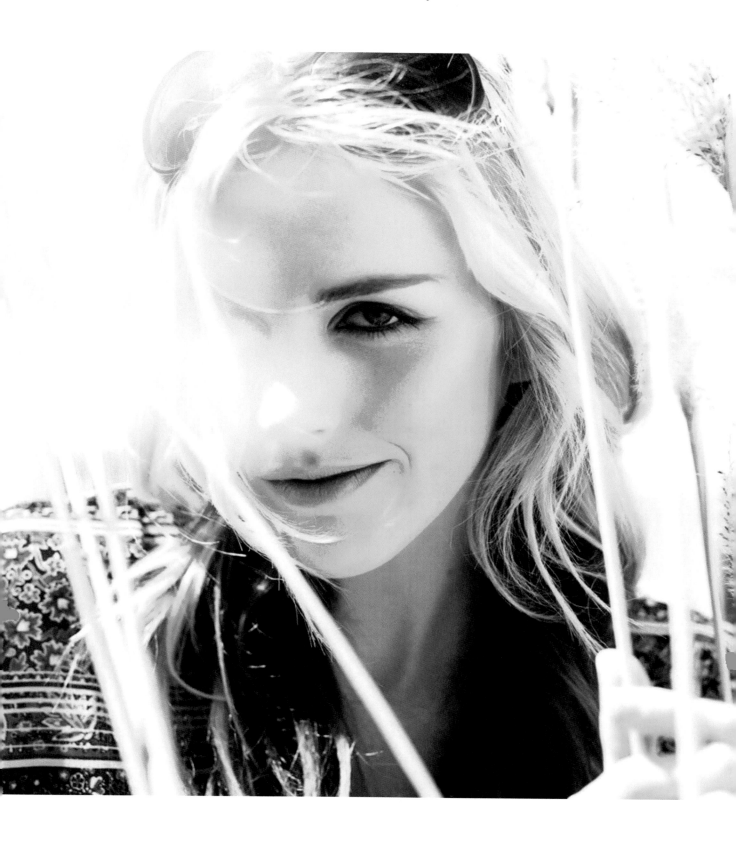

Bridal Makeup

Wedding day makeup should enhance your most beautiful features.

On your wedding day you want to look like yourself only a more beautiful version of you. Your wedding day makeup should be as natural looking as possible, but it should also emphasize your features so you look flawless in photographs. But most important you want your face to look smooth, even and flawless and remember your wedding day is not the day to experiment with trendy or glitzy new makeup applications.

Applying your bridal makeup depends on both the theme and time of your wedding but more important it is about capturing the essence of you. An evening wedding can be slightly more dramatic with sultry smoky eyes and bolder shadows. A perfect time for tight lining the eyes with a black or dark brown eye liner. This will give depth and dimension in the shadows of an evening wedding.

The most important ingredient in flawless wedding day makeup no matter what time of the day you have your ceremony is using quality products that suit your skin type and skin tone. Every bride deserves to look flawless on her wedding day. So preparing for this day and practicing your makeup skills will make the day of the wedding go smoothly and run with very little stress. Remember tensions run high on the big day, but you can ease the stress by remaining cool and confident in your skills this will give you the best bridal face ever. And don't let anyone distract you from the creation of your wedding day makeup application. If at all possible do your makeup in an environment away from distractions and excited friends and family.

Daytime Bridal Makeup

Daytime bridal makeup should be flawless and minimal with lighter eye shades and rosy lips that enhance your look to create a more beautiful version of you. Your daytime bridal look should emphasize your glowing cheeks, romantic eyes and luscious lips for the most foolproof and timeless bridal beauty. To get the most from your wedding day look you will want to appear timeless for your wedding photos capturing you with glowing beauty. No matter what your style is, you will want your daytime make to give you ethereal beauty and a timeless look. Applying your makeup is a gift that very few women give themselves, a quiet time to gaze into your own eyes and begin wrapping the package of you that your groom is going to receive, a gift no greater than that is required.

You will want to apply your makeup before putting on the wedding gown unless it must go over the head, in this case, use button up top to cover and protect your gown.

Evening Bridal Makeup

Evening bridal makeup should be a bit heavier with darker hues to enhance the eyes and lips, you can apply heavier highlighting to overcome low lights and it is always a good idea to apply deeper tones to the lips to get them to stand out. Evening wedding makeup should emphasize your beautiful features without overpower them. Evening weddings are meant for romance so be sure not to try out any trendy new looks that you might find in a nightclub, stick to traditional makeup that emphasizes your beauty and doesn't cover it up.

"The beauty of a woman must be seen from in her eyes, because that is the doorway to her heart, the place where love resides" -Audrey Hepburn

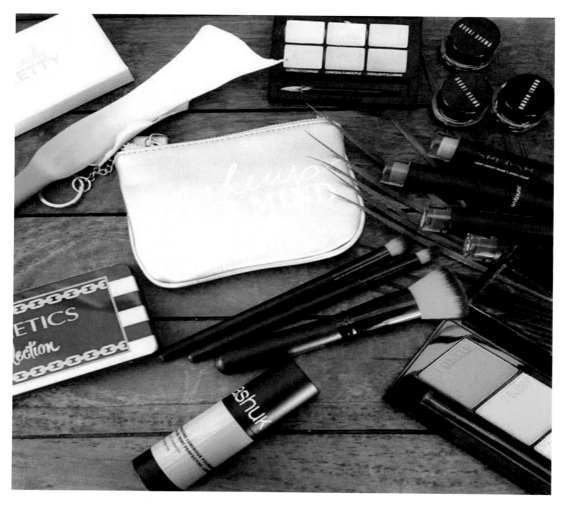

10 Step Bridal Makeup Application
Your guide to flawless wedding day makeup.

Step 1: Primer

The most important step to achieving a lasting wedding day makeup look is to use a quality primer that is lightweight, goes on smooth, and applies easily to the face, neck and the lids of the eyes. Primer has two objectives, to keep your makeup in place all day and to minimize the appearance of fine lines and large pores. Your primer will act as a skin spackle keeping your makeup in place all day and concealing those little face flaws no one else needs to see.

Be sure to test at least three different brands of primers to find the one that works best with your skin type. There are many different primers on the market, you can get them from the drugstore, cosmetics counters, designer cosmetic stores, direct sales makeup companies or even online from your favorite makeup company. No matter where you decide to get your primer or what brand you decide to use make sure it works well with your skin type and stays in place all day. Don't be afraid to ask for samples when you're out makeup shopping.

Primer is essential to your makeup look and getting the right primer for your skin type will prove to be one of the most important steps in your 10 step bridal makeup application.

Primer is the bond and the spackle that creates a flawless finish for your makeup application to sit upon and get the lasting results you need for a long wearing makeup application. You will need to test out your primer and find the one that works well with your skin and can hold up to the elements as well as the human contact you will be having throughout your wedding and reception.

Primer is a critical step and one that cant be missed. We recommend using a face primer as well as an eyelid primer. The eye primer is made for the thin skin of the eyes and helps to keep your eye makeup from creasing.

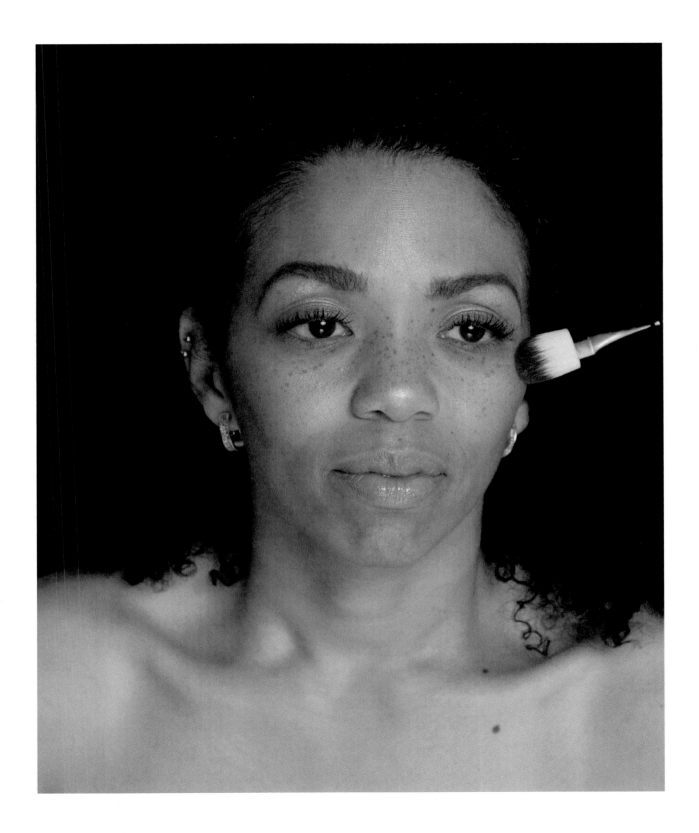

Step 2: Correct and Conceal

Concealers and correctors are your bridal makeup secret weapons and correcting those tiny flaws on your face is essential to a flawless finish.

Correctors are exactly what they claim to be and they are necessary to erase those tiny flaws on your face that can show through under your foundation if not taken care of before your foundation is applied. A corrector is used to cover acne spots, scars, and redness on the face or purple hues that often appear under our eyes or on our eyelids. Your corrector colors are usually green, yellow or peach. Green is used to hide red spots from acne. Yellow is used to correct purple hues under the eyes or on the eyelids and pink or peach colored corrector can be used on scars or to neutralize discoloration.

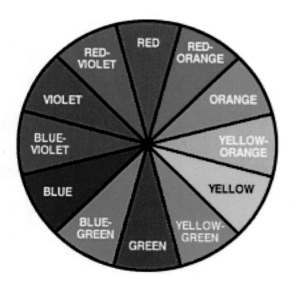

Use the color wheel to gage what color you need to do a color correction.

Example: If you have redness from acne or rosacea use the opposite color on the color wheel to even out and neutralize the redness.

Concealers are more to brighten your face and to cover the correctors you have just applied. I recommend you apply your concealer after you have applied your foundation but you choose the time to apply that best suits your needs.

Start with a beige or yellow concealer one color lighter than your skin tone under the eyes and create a V shape that runs from under your eye down to the top of your cheek and blend it with upward and outward strokes to the outer corner of your eye.

This technique needs to be blended well and must not appear harsh in its finished state.

Learning how to use correctors and concealers are essential in your makeup routine and once applied they should be blended well on the edges of the application. Correcting and concealing takes practice and patience and an understanding of the flaws you want to hide and the areas of the face you want to enhance.

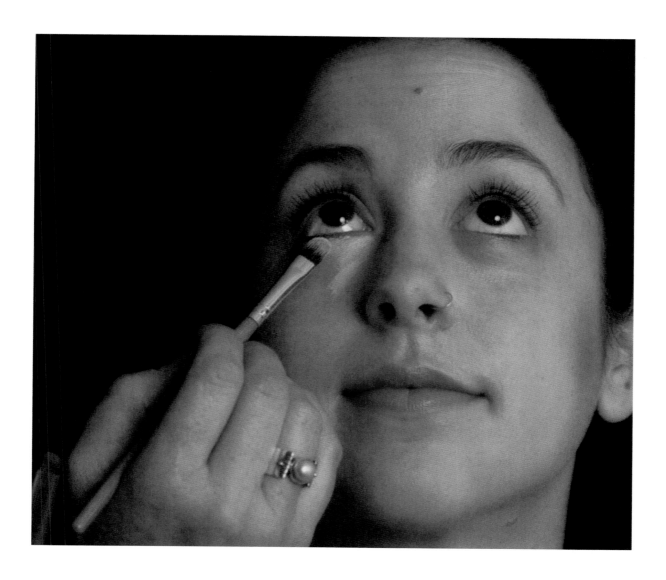

Step 3: Foundation

Finding the correct color and consistency of foundation is a vital step in your makeup application. You want a foundation that is the exact color of your skin tone and at the same time has the right consistency to cover your flaws but light enough to not look over done. The right foundation should give a flawless finish that lasts all day, looks luminous, and is sweat proof.

Foundation Strip Test

One of the first steps in foundation is finding the right color for your skin. This is a step you will want to make sure you do not skip. Your foundation should be an exact match of your skin and blend seamlessly into your chin and neck. Make sure to do a foundation strip test. Our model has three stripes on her face and one is almost invisible.

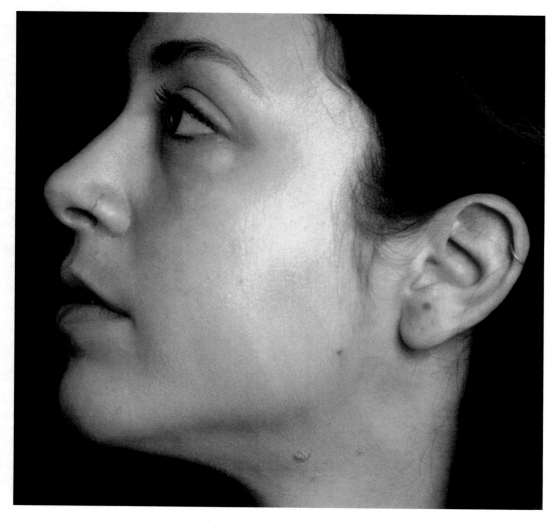

Applying Foundation

☐ Apply foundation to your face using your fingertips covering all areas of the face, this technique warms the product and makes it easy to apply.

☐ Once you have covered your face, neck and chin use a stiff flat brush to gently blend the product over the entire face, and down the neck giving it an airbrushed finished.

☐ Check that you have blended well into the sides of the face, the chin and the neck so there are no harsh lines of demarcation.

☐ Give a final check to make sure your finish is flawless.

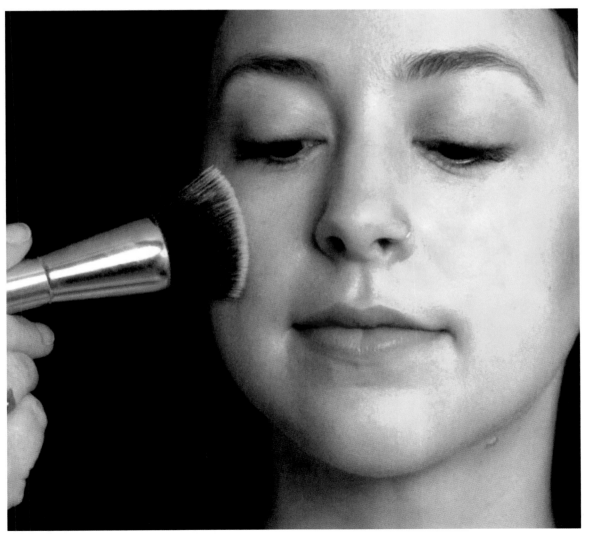

5 Rules of Foundation

Can you get a perfect and flawless makeup foundation? Can you really achieve flawless looking skin and still look like you're wearing nothing at all?

With a few simple rules to follow you can get the flawless foundation you are looking for! Just take the time to follow these 5 simple rules of foundation and you will get the flawless results you are looking for.

1. Choose the right product.
2. Know what product works best with your skin type (mineral powder foundations, liquid foundations, cream foundations).
3. Choose the right color.
4. Apply with a brush blending technique.
5. Set with a spray or setting powder.

Foundation is a critical step in your wedding day makeup application and your color should be well established long before the wedding day. But with that said be sure to bring two shades of color, we often times get a little sun and our skin tone can change. It is not unusual to blend two colors together to get a perfect color match for your skin.

Foundation Options

Powder: Usually a mineral foundation that gives full coverage and works well with oily and youthful skin.

Liquid: Usually leaves a dewy finish that can give you full coverage or a more translucent coverage depending on it's consistency and the application it was designed for. It is perfect for dry skin and older skin.

Cream: A perfect option for giving full coverage to problem skin, cream foundations have a thicker consistency and go on like a liquid and are best applied with beauty blenders or sponges, but remember to use your foundation brush to blend in the hairline and under the chin and neck to give an airbrushed finish.

It really doesn't matter which type of foundation you use, just be sure to use the right color that's best suited for your skin type and one that matches your skin tone perfectly.

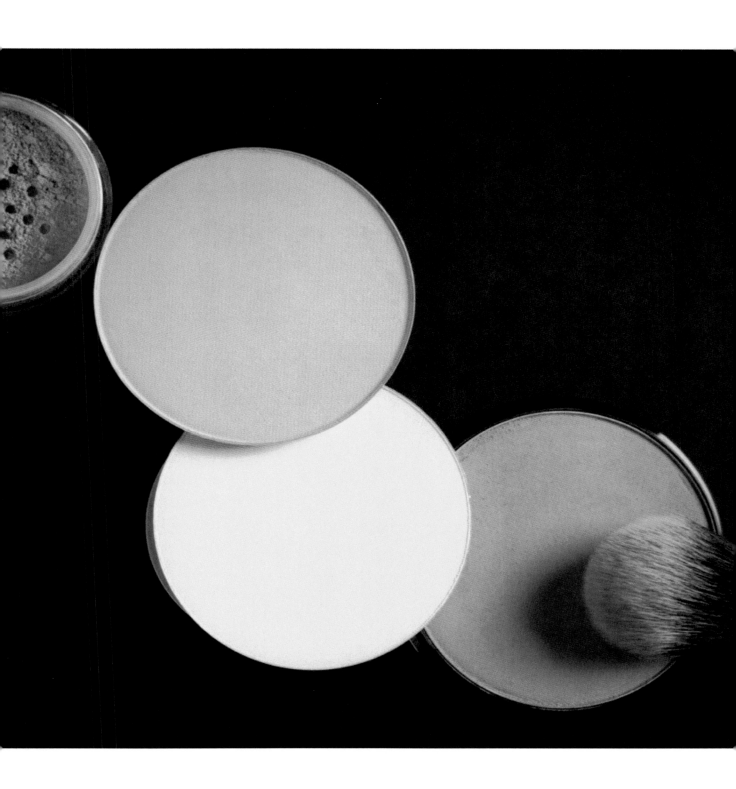

Step 4: Setting Powders

Setting your concealer and foundation is an important step in your makeup application and one you don't want to miss. Use a quality translucent powder or a yellow toned translucent powder on your face and neck to give you a shine free look that will ensure when your photos arrive your face will have a perfect finish. Setting your foundation can make or break your wedding day photos. Remember your wedding day photos will be with you a lifetime and you want them to be perfect.

☐ Use a large puffy brush.

☐ Choose a quality setting powered in a translucent or yellow toned shade.

☐ Be very sparing with your setting powder you don't want your makeup to look caked.

☐ If you are an older bride I suggest not using any powder on your face, powders tend to settle in fine lines and is not a kind product for a flawless finish.

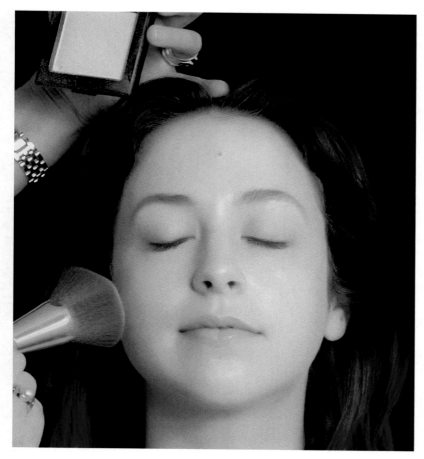

If you are an older bride stay away from powder products, they tend to enhance fine lines, wrinkles and large pores. Instead opt for a setting spray.

Step 5: Contour & Bronze

Your wedding day is not the day for heavy contouring or loads of bronzer, it's an opportunity to enhance your best features by giving depth and dimension as well as a natural lift to your face. The same applies to using a bronzer which gives your skin a kiss of sun.

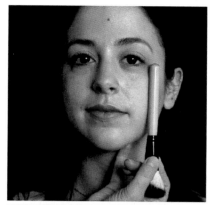

Your contour color should be two shades darker than your natural skin tone but not to dark that it will make your face look sculpted and un-natural.

Contouring Rich Skin Tones

There is no need to contour rich or dark olive skin tones you were blessed with rich skin that needs no contouring. We will talk further on how you can give depth to your skin tone by using cream highlighters and lighter concealers.

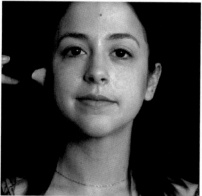

Contouring

☐ Your cheek contour should not come in further than the outer corner of your eye. Use your contour brush and check where your contour should end.

☐ Use a contour shade just a bit darker than your skin tone and apply just below each cheek bone, sweeping out toward the hair.

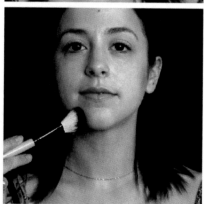

☐ If necessary on a large forehead contour along the hairline to slim the face.

☐ Slim down a large chin by placing a fine dust of contour around the chin enhancing the end of the chin bone.

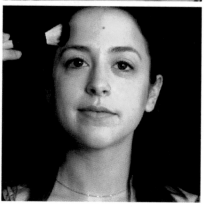

If you feel like you need to slim down a sagging chin area, use your contour just under the jawline giving the illusion of shadow to mask a sagging chin area.

Bronzing

☐ Apply bronzer to the chest area if you are wearing a strapless or low cut gown. Be sure to not over do it with your bronzer and choose a shade that brightens not a shade that can make your skin look dirty.

☐ Bronzer can also be applied to the forehead and on the cheeks or anywhere that the sunlight would hit on the face or anywhere that needs a kiss of sun. Do not overdo the bronzer it can quickly darken the face and neck very quickly.

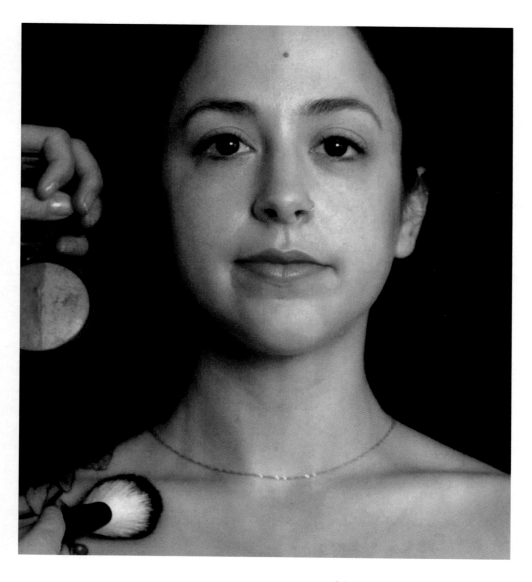

Your bronzer should be brightening with a shimmer to the base, you want to look like the sun has kissed you from above.

There are many bronzers on the market so be sure to pick one that gives light to your face and neck.

Step 6: Blush

For a fresh and luminous glow use a two-step blush application. Blush when applied correctly wakes the face up and adds warmth.

☐ Apply a light natural shade of blush to the cheekbones moving in an upward swirl to the hairline.

☐ Next apply a brighter pink or peach applied just to the apples of the cheek then lightly blended into the natural shade to bring the two colors together. This will brighten your face for a realistic blushing bride finish.

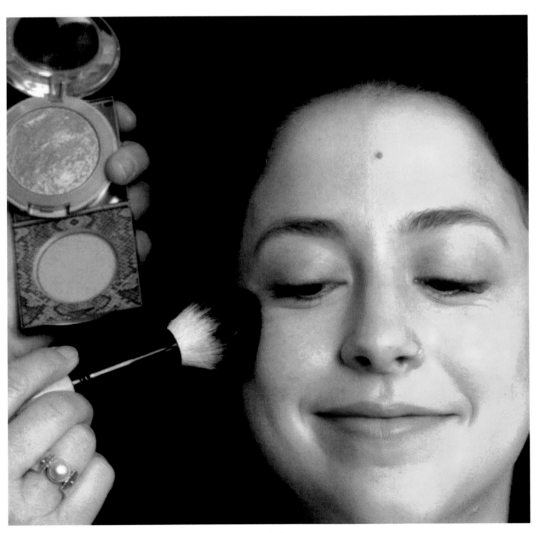

Step 7: Showcasing Your Eyes

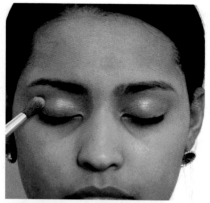

Showcasing your eyes is the most challenging application of the entire DIY makeup application but if you follow these easy to apply steps you will master the technique very quickly. Your wedding day is not the time to have heavy smoky eyes or to test out trendy new looks. Your wedding day is about an ethereal look that enhances your natural beauty. Avoid bright or dark colors, stick to pinks, peaches, light grays or charcoal.

Shadowing Steps

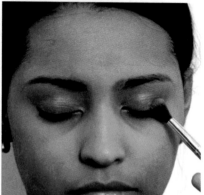

- ☐ Apply primer to the eyelids.

- ☐ Apply a light beige to the entire eye lid.

- ☐ Apply a pink or peach to the lower lid stopping at the crease line.

- ☐ Apply a charcoal or dark brown to the outer corner of the lower lid in the crease line, blending 1/3 of the way toward the center and then to the lash line 1/3 of the way in. Blend well.

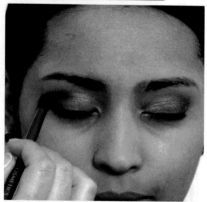

- ☐ Apply a shimmer beige or light silver to the inner corner of the lower lid and just below the brow on the brow bone.

The secret to great eye shadow application is using quality products with a high pigment content, then you will need to blend well to get a seamless look of each color coming together.

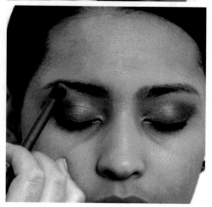

Showcasing your eyes is important, you want your eyes to look alluring and romantic on your wedding day, but try not to overdo the look, keep it simple and flawless.

Eye Liner

Eye liner doesn't have to be difficult it can be challenging at first to understand how to hold your brush and how to get a smooth line but with practice and quality brushes eye lining can be easy to achieve.

Try the tight lining technique for your eyeliner to showcase the eyes, this technique is much easier to apply with damp eye shadow using a liner brush or very small stiff flat brush. Don't be afraid to test out liner products. This technique can be done with powder shadows, liner pencil or lose pigments.

- Line the upper lash line with a dark charcoal, dark brown or light black.
- Line the lower lash line with the same color coming in only 3/4 of the way.
- Soften the liner by smudging it with a bigger flat brush.

Eye lining is a skill that requires a lot of practice this technique used on our model is achieved by using a black eye shadow and wetting our brush to create a thick paste then applying the paste with a fine lining brush to the upper lash line and the lower lash line and to the upper inside lash line. You can darken the look be adding a gel liner over the top of the upper lash line when you have completed your entire eye makeup application.

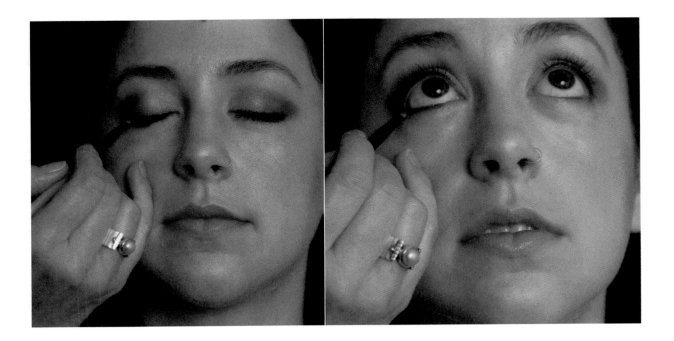

Brows

Defining the eye brows will create a natural frame for the face and make eyes pop in your wedding photos. Be sure to use the correct color brow powder or brow pencil to fill-in brows, we suggest a two-color brow process to get a natural look.

☐ Apply the first color the same as your natural brow color or hair color to the lower brow line and move in hair like strokes to the out brow

☐ Use the lighter color to the inside corner of the brow using hair like strokes and to the upper hairline to give the brow depth and definition.

Your brows complete the face and without some type of enhancement or correction you can leave your face looking unfinished. Brow products come in pencils, powders and even gels.

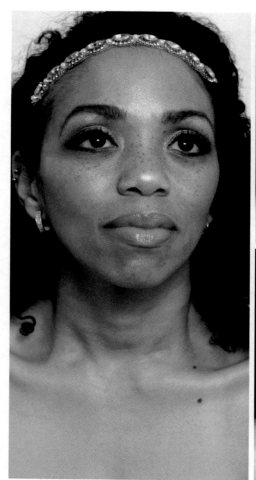
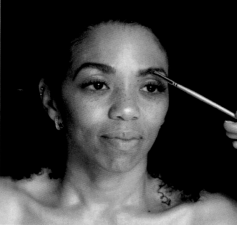
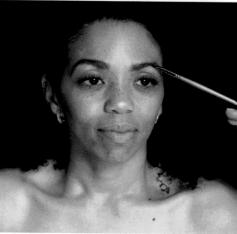

No matter what product you use on your brows always apply it with hair like strokes during the application.

Eye Brow Shaping

Eye brow shaping is a skill you will develop over time but the basic shape is as follows:

- ☐ The brow starts on the inner corner of the nose. Use a thin long brush or your eye brow pencil to gage the starting point of the brow. Place a small dot for you to start your brow line.

- ☐ The arch of the brow should can be determined by holding your brow pencil at an angle coming up from the nose and running through the pupil o the eye. Place a small dot to gage where the high point of the brow should be.

- ☐ The outer corner of the brow can be determined by placing the brow pencil at a wide angle coming our from the corner of the nose and running on the outer corner of the eye. Place a small dot the gage where the eye brow should finish.

- ☐ Fill in the brow with small hair like strokes.

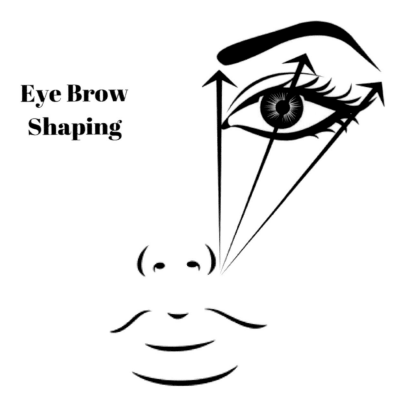

Eye Brow Shaping

The eyebrow makeup application completes all makeup looks and is a must when it comes to the 10 step bridal makeup application. No face looks complete without well shaped brows filled in with a color the same shade as your hair.

Lashes

Enhancing your lashes will be the final step of your eye makeup application and we recommend getting lash extensions if you can afford it or don't want to fuss with your lashes or use fiber lash mascara if you can find it topped off with black waterproof mascara in case you spill a few tears!

False Lashes

If you want more pop, the easiest false lash technique for a novice is to use individual lashes that come with three lashes on each band. These lashes can be applied to the outer 1/3 corner of your lash line after your mascara application. This is so much easier than learning to apply false lashes which can be a challenge for even the most qualified makeup artist. The last thing you want to happen on your wedding day is to have a lash strip come loose, this will mean pulling off both lash stripes leaving you without the long lush lashes you desire. You can get these individual lashes at any beauty supply store and even at high end retailers. Be sure to get the black glue used to apply the lashes so you don't have white dots on your lash line from the glue.

Lash Application

Step 1: Choose the length of lash you want to use.

Step 2: Apply the lash glue to the end of the lash.

Step 3: Wait one minute to let the glue setup.

Step 4: Apply the lash onto your lash line.

Step 5: Set the lash by pushing down on the tip of the lash until it blends with your own lashes.

Step 6: Apply the lashes to just the 1/3 outer corner of your lash line.

Step: Wait a few minutes for the lashes to firm up and dry into place.

Lashes are very important and need to be well thought out in advance of your wedding day. If you can afford to get lash extensions and they are available in your area indulge in this even if its just a one time splurge. If not then practice the lash technique you will use on your wedding day it will matter at the end of the day.

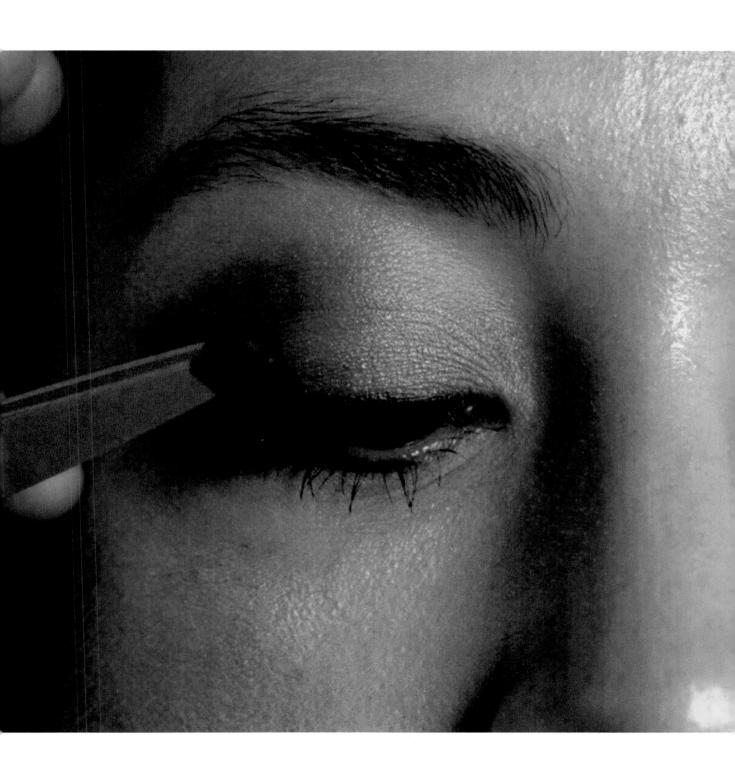

Step 8: Lips

Lip sculpting has become the newest rage in makeup and although we do not recommend trend makeup in the bridal makeup application process we do think using this technique on your wedding day is a great way to give you the romantic lips you are looking for. Achieving flawless lips is all about creating a plump and pouty look for a more romantic appearance to bring your lips forward for your wedding day pictures.

Your lip products will be the first makeup to disappear during your wedding day so using our three step application will ensure a longer lasting look, but even with that said, make sure you have your wedding day lip color on hand to refresh your look throughout the day. Give your mini bridal makeup kit to your bridesmaid or a family member to keep in case you need to refresh your lips.

You will want to make sure you top off your lips right before you do your photo shoot. Use your lipstick throughout the day and keep it handy in an easy to access location.

Ask your photographer if the color of lipstick you have chosen will work well with the pictures they are going to take.

When it comes to bridal makeup your lips matter a great deal.

Lip Sculpting

☐ Line your lips with a color one shade darker than your natural lip color.

☐ Line the corners of your lips one third of the way in with the liner color.

☐ Fill in the area inside the lip liner with a shade that is exactly the same color as your natural lips with a lip liner pencil or lip stain (we used the Mally Duo Lip Pencil).

☐ Top off your lips with a lipstick in pink, peach or plum or use your favorite lip gloss in a bright shade that pops to give your lips a lux look.

Natural lips with a pop of color are the secret to lip sculpting.

Starting with a natural base and building out the corners of the lips with a shade one color darker to give them definition, then topping your lips off with a blast of color and sealing it in with a gloss or lipstick to maintain it's longevity.

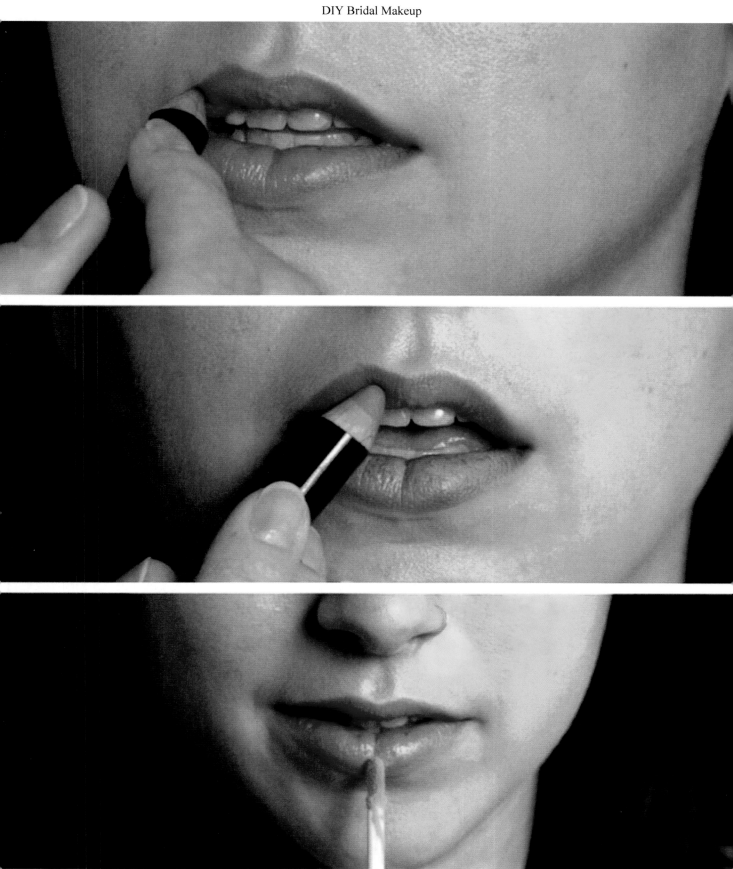

Lip Colors

Your wedding lipstick shades can range in color from nudes, pinks, plums, sand tones and even coral, no matter what color you choose check to make sure it looks good with the dress you wear and is well paired with your skin tone.

Remember your lips need to be bright and sunny but not over dramatic.

Bridal Lipstick Colors

Getting the right color lips for your skin tone can be crucial in your wedding day photos.

Fair Skin: Nude, Pink, Mauve

Medium: Rose, Pink, Mauve

Olive: Peach, Coral, Dark Rose

Deep: Peach, Red, Coral

Choose the lip color you feel the most comfortable wearing and remember your wedding day is not the day to step to far out of your comfort zone and try new or trendy shades. It is a time for subtle, soft, full, and romantically kissable lips. Your lips will be exposed to many variables on your wedding day and you want to feel and look like yourself.

There are many options for wedding day lip colors.

- ☐ Lip Pencil
- ☐ Lipstick
- ☐ Lip Gloss
- ☐ Lip Stain
- ☐ Lip Balm

Use this handy bridal lip chart to help you determine the best color for your skin tone.

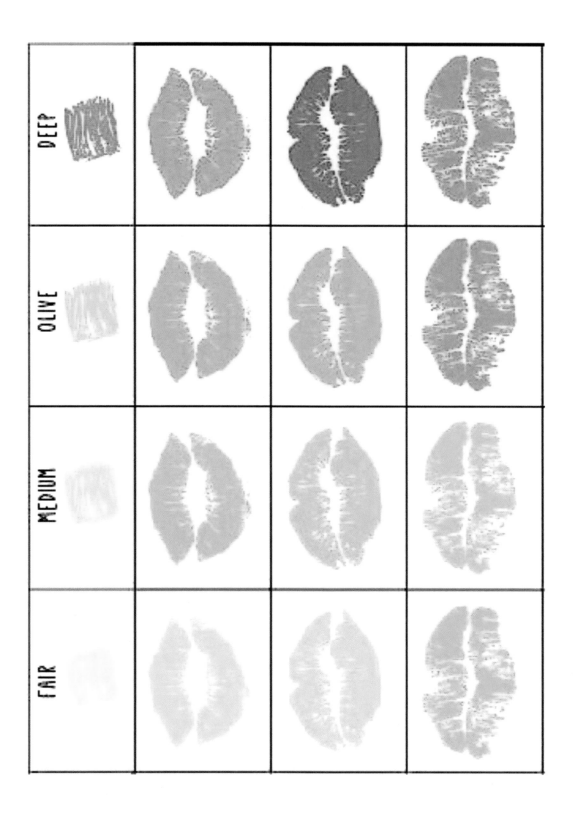

Step 9: Highlight & Brighten

Highlighting in a makeup application is a relatively new concept in the world of makeup but it has been a well kept secret of professional makeup artists. Makeup artists have been highlighting their clients for years and understand the importance of this step in the makeup application. Makeup artists know the importance of highlighting to create more light on the face and to brighten up a flawless makeup application.

Highlighting your face at the end of your makeup application gives you a shimmering glamorous glow and will enhance your wedding day photos with the illusion of perfect lighting.

1. Apply a powder highlighter below the brow, on the top of the brow bone, and on the top of your cheek bone over the top of your blusher.

2. Apply your powder highlighter to the cupids bow on the top of your upper lip.

Highlighting is the secret weapon of celebrities who use the camera as their best friend to draw attention to their faces.

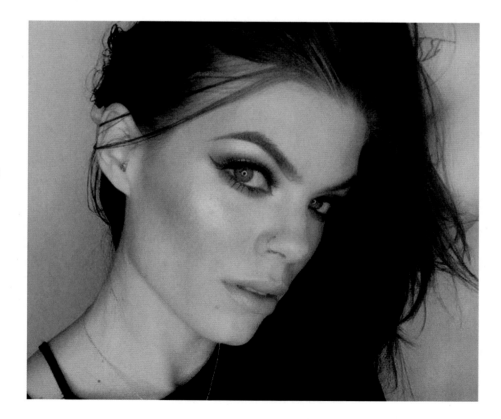

Step 10: Maintain Your Glow

The final step of success in your bridal makeup look will be to keep your skin looking fresh and dewy all day, this will require diligence on your part throughout the wedding day.

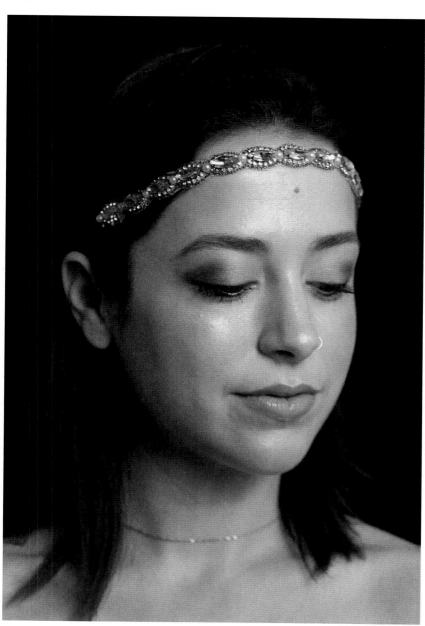

If you were unable to set your foundation and concealer with a setting powder you will now need to spritz your face with a setting spray.

Hydration will be very important throughout the day to keep your skin plump and radiant. Dehydrated skin when left unattended will begin to appear sallow and will enhance fine lines. Most brides get so caught up in all the excitement of the day that they tend to forget to keep their bodies hydrated. Drinking water throughout the day and evening is the final step in keeping your gorgeous makeup flawless.

Face Shapes

The shape of your face may not seem like an important element when doing your bridal makeup application but for certain face shapes applying contour products and eye makeup can be a challenge.

So to get the best makeup application on your wedding day you must understand how and where to apply your contour makeup as well as your blush.

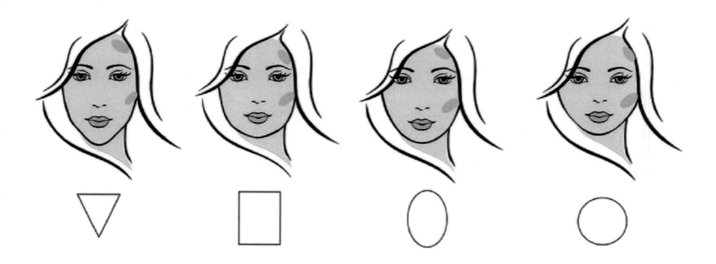

The most common face shapes are triangle. Square, oval and round, each one has its one uniqueness and each one needs to be approached uniquely with your contouring, bronzing and blush applications.

Face Shapes

Triangle Face: This face needs very light or no contouring at all since contouring is meant to give depth and dimension to your face, and as you can see the triangle face has that already built in. You may want to add a very small amount of contouring under the cheekbone to decrease the length of this face and to the upper hairline to give fullness to the face.

Square Face: The square face is also a face that has lots of depth and dimension built in but needs contouring under the cheekbone in a thin line creating depth and to the upper hairline right above the eyebrow adding length to the face.

Oval Face: The oval face has the gift of length built in and needs less under cheek contouring than other face shapes. You can add a small amount of contouring under the cheekbone and higher on the forehead hairline to shorten this face shape.

Round Face: The round face has the cheeks we all desire but needs depth and dimension to bring the best features of the face forward. Contour heavier under the cheekbone of the round face and along the hairline, keep the contour away from the upper forehead. We want to give length to the round face so keep the contour closer to the hairline in an upward line.

Your face shape is unique to you and although you can't change it's shape you can change the depth and give the illusion of dimension using contouring and blush techniques.

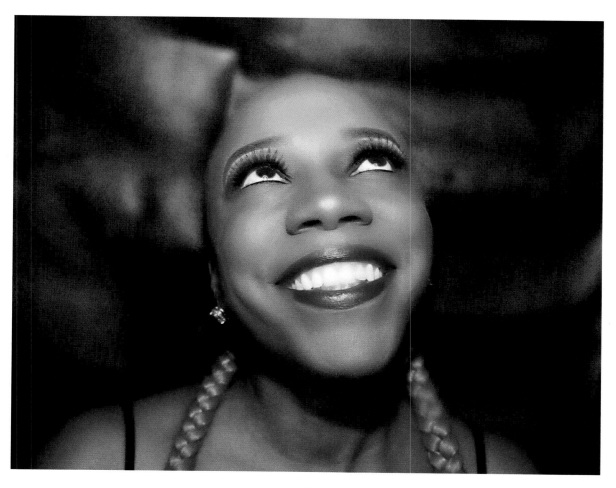

Bridal Makeup Face Chart

Products are key to your wedding day makeup success.

Keeping a list of the products you have tested and love in your bridal makeup application is important as you decide which products you are going to use. Using a face chart can guide you when you are packing your wedding day makeup kit. It is also important if you decide to have a professional makeup artist do your makeup, they will then have a guide to follow of the products and placement of your makeup on your wedding day.

Bridal Makeup Product Chart

Primer:

Foundation:

Concealer:

Contour:

Bronzer:

Blush:

Eye Shadows:

Eye Liner:

Brows:

Mascara:

Lip Liner:

Lip Stick:

Lip Gloss:

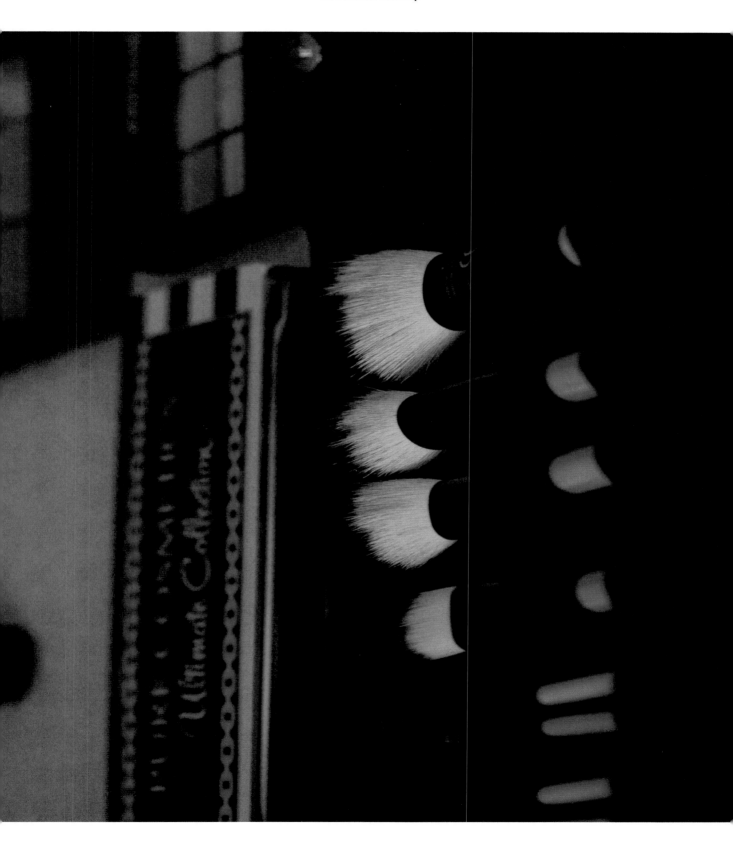

The 7 Day Bridal Beauty Countdown

With so many last minute things to consider we know this 7 day beauty countdown is probably already on your list of things to do, but if by chance you need a little extra guidance here is our 7 day beauty countdown.

7 days before your wedding is a good time to get those ends trimmed on your hair.

6 days before your wedding is a good time to get those underarms, lips, eyebrows, and legs waxed.

5 days before your wedding you may want to apply a very light shade of self tanner, but beware most photographers discourage self tanners because they tend to look orange in photos.

4 days before your wedding treat yourself to a pedicure or a massage. This relaxing time may help to calm you as you head into the craziness of last minute wedding planning.

3 days before your wedding is the perfect time to give yourself a manicure or run out and get a professional manicure.

2 days before your wedding make sure to start drinking plenty of water to hydrate your body and face. Water is your secret weapon to a beautiful and glowing you on your wedding day.

1 day before your wedding is a good time to go for a walk or take a yoga class and maybe ask your groom-to-be out for a quiet walk together and reconnect during a time of great stress on both of you.

Your wedding day has arrived and this is a good day to let others do their jobs and take the one hour of designated and quiet time to apply your wedding day makeup. Remember you are the gift to your groom and today you will be wrapping that gift in the beauty of you.

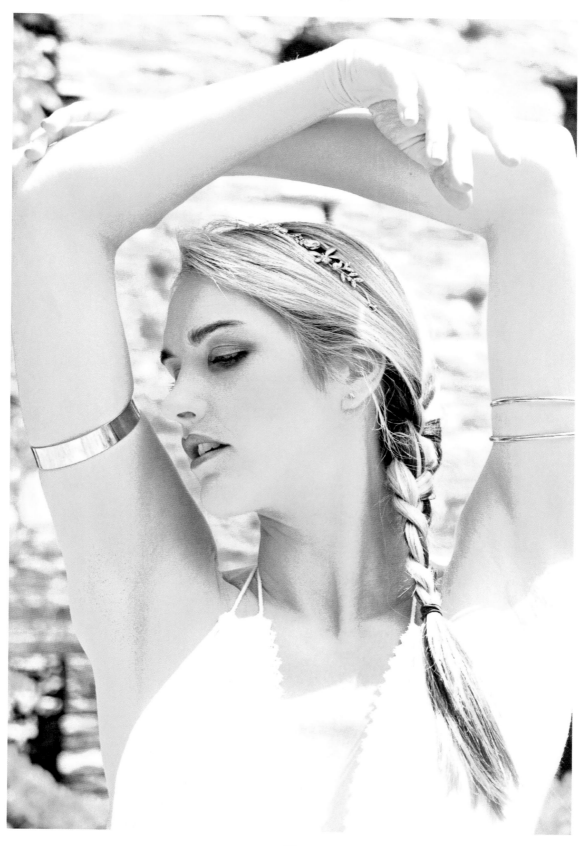

History of DIY Bridal Makeup
Doing one's own wedding day makeup is a long standing tradition.

For centuries women have been doing their own wedding day makeup or letting family and friends prepare them for their special day. Throughout history the bride has enhanced her features in the beautification process for her groom to present him with the most beautiful version of herself. The gift of beautification on the wedding day has been a tradition in almost every culture for centuries and that tradition is still a part of weddings in every culture in the world today. The gift is in the process of preparing oneself to be received into the heart and arms of ones groom.

For centuries the Greek wedding tradition has been for the brides maid of honor and her closest friends to dress her and prepare her hair, makeup and body on her wedding day. This intimate ritual is a custom that dates back many centuries and is still in practice today.

Traditional Japanese brides for centuries typically wear red lipstick, with a more pale looking makeup application topped of with an elaborate headpiece that emphasizes her stature. The red lipstick signifies passion and love and is the gift of the bride to her groom.

In the Indian or Hindu tradition you will find the bride has been prepared with elaborate eye makeup applications in jewel toned shadows highlighted with a colorful gown adorned with bright and shiny jewels and often accompanied by colorful flower adornments. The emphasis on the eyes creates a seductive look that is enhanced by her olive skin tone and traditional bridal gown. In this traditional style wedding you will find bright flowers and beautiful colors everywhere. Henna is one of the many beautiful body beautification traditions that have been a part of this culture for centuries. Although not a makeup application it is a form of body beautification that is an enhancement that signifies the special day in an ancient tradition.

Wedding day beautification happens in almost every culture in the world and often these enhancements are performed by the bride or the brides closest friends and family. It is a time to reflect and celebrate the bride and her beauty and then present this beatification to her groom and the many guests at her wedding day.

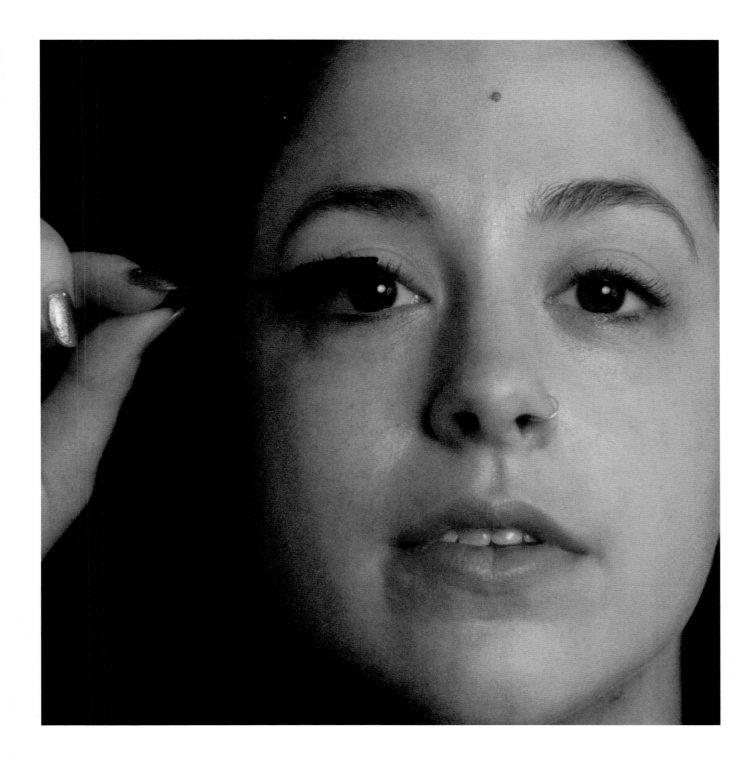

DIY Bridal Makeup Workshops

We teach beauty, you create beautiful.

We are fortunate to bring you our 10 step bridal makeup application in this guidebook and thrilled you have taken the first step in creating a flawless wedding day makeup look. But if you want a more in depth guide or want to watch our tutorial videos we have created an easy step-by-step online workshop, we encourage you to head on over to our online DIY Bridal Makeup workshop at womeningear.com then click on Bridal Makeup Course.

This workshop is filled with bonus features, such as an in depth lash application tutorial video, the four color eye shadow application tutorial video, and a guide to help you figure out your skin type and your exact skin tone. We created this online workshop as a bonus to give you the bride access to our video tutorials right up to your wedding day. This online class will help you to perfect your bridal makeup application skills and teaches you how to get the best products to use in your makeup application.

You can access our online School of Makeup Artistry and our DIY Bridal Makeup Class at womeningear.com.

We also are fortunate to teach bridal makeup workshops all over the United States and Europe, you can see our events schedule on our website and attend one of our live workshops where we teach you the 10 step bridal makeup application in a group setting. These live classes give you a front row seat to see Keisha and I or one of our trained instructors teaching our bridal makeup techniques.

Each attendee at our live classes receives a swag bag filled with makeup goodies and a signed copy of our DIY Bridal Makeup guidebook as well as access to our online Bridal Makeup Course. We encourage you to head over to our website and check out the events section to see if we are going to be in your city this coming year.

We look forward to meeting you on our tour across the United States and Europe.

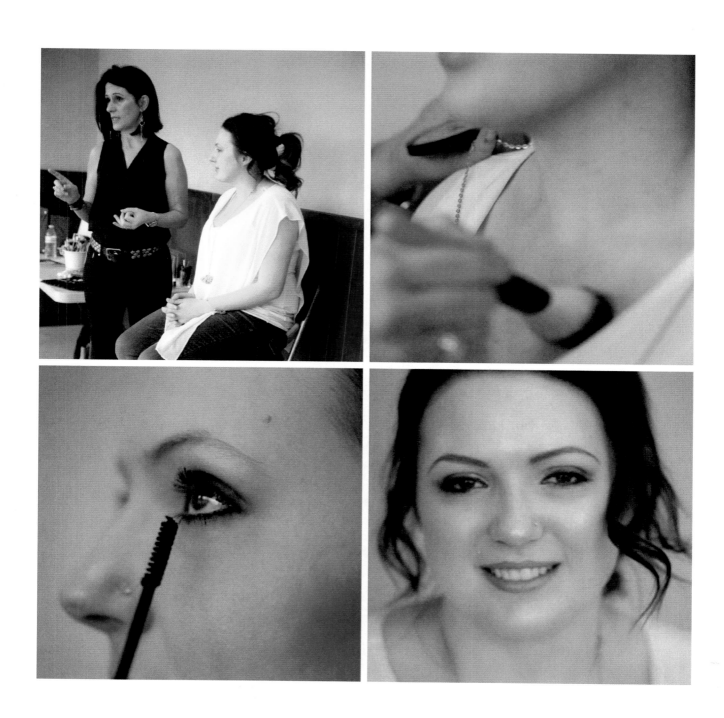

Acknowledgments

Alone we are smart, together we are brilliant.

There is no way a single person can write a book or complete a training manual that gives value to others without the help of many people collaborating together to make it a reality. This book is no different and I am blessed to have an incredible business partner, a supportive family, and a wonderful husband who believes that if we apply ourselves and follow through on our dreams anything is possible.

I would first like to acknowledge you the reader for taking the time to read this guide book and for knowing that yes you can achieve flawless wedding day makeup on your own, it is in that belief of yourself that all things in life are accomplished.

I want to say thank you to my co-author and collaborator on the DIY Bridal Makeup book Keisha Garrett for taking a leap of faith with me and spending countless hours taking photographs, applying makeup, teaching workshops and driving hundreds of miles to make this book a reality. You are truly the hardest working MUA/Photographer in all of Virginia.

To the beautiful and talented Brittany Walker, your many contributions to this book as well as all your contributions to the online makeup courses offered at The School of Makeup Artistry are what has made it so successful. Your talent with makeup and creating flawless makeup videos is one of the reasons I felt so inspired to write this book, your artistic talents never cease to amaze me.

I want to thank my beautiful daughter Josha Gleich who spent countless hours editing this book, without your support nothing in my life is possible. Everyday you take the time for me and share the joy of your life as if you were living right next door instead of 3000 miles away. Thank you for giving me guidance, your knowledge and grasp of makeup and the application of makeup is a gift I cherish.

To my better half Rob Thomas, you have given me the best days of my life and I am honored and humbled to call you my husband. Your support of me and my business endeavors has never wavered, even when I made wrong steps and expensive errors you encouraged me to continue to pursue my dreams. Your saying, that someday you want to leave your high stress career and just follow me around carrying my briefcase and supporting my business still makes me laugh and inspires me to push through even when it's tough. I am me because of you.

To my family and friends, you are my tribe and without your love and support I would not have been brave enough or felt confident enough to write a book about that which I am so passionate about.

To all the students, it was an honor teach every one of you over the past seven years and I want to thank you for always listening to what I had to impart and for asking all the right questions. Each question asked from you brought not only knowledge to you but brought knowledge to me. I ask that each of you continue to pursue your dreams and live the life you were given to the fullest, honing your talents and bettering your skills will truly make you the best in your industry

To Bobbi Brown, who has no idea the influence she has had on my life and my journey into the world of makeup and beauty. Your makeup instruction showed me that enhancing the natural beauty of a woman is so much more important than covering up her best features. The Bobbi Brown Makeup Manual has been my makeup bible for many years and I still refer to it today for guidance when I need it.

I may teach beauty but you my friends create beautiful.

Toni Thomas, xoxo

Credits

Collaboration is the key to everything.

Thank you to the contributors and collaborators of this book, you made it possible for Keisha and I to bring this guidebook to all the brides-to-be looking for a way to do their own wedding day makeup and achieve a flawless finish. Without your participation this book would not have been possible.

Photographers

Keisha Garrett

Ryan Hicks

Toni Thomas

Rodney Valentine

Nick Kalivretenos

Models

Brittany Walker

Nikki Weede

Kelly Reddin

Shanica Campbell

Amber Hensley

Cynthia Vasquez

Editor

Josha Gleich

Other Sources

Pinterest

Canva

Collaboration is the key to everything!

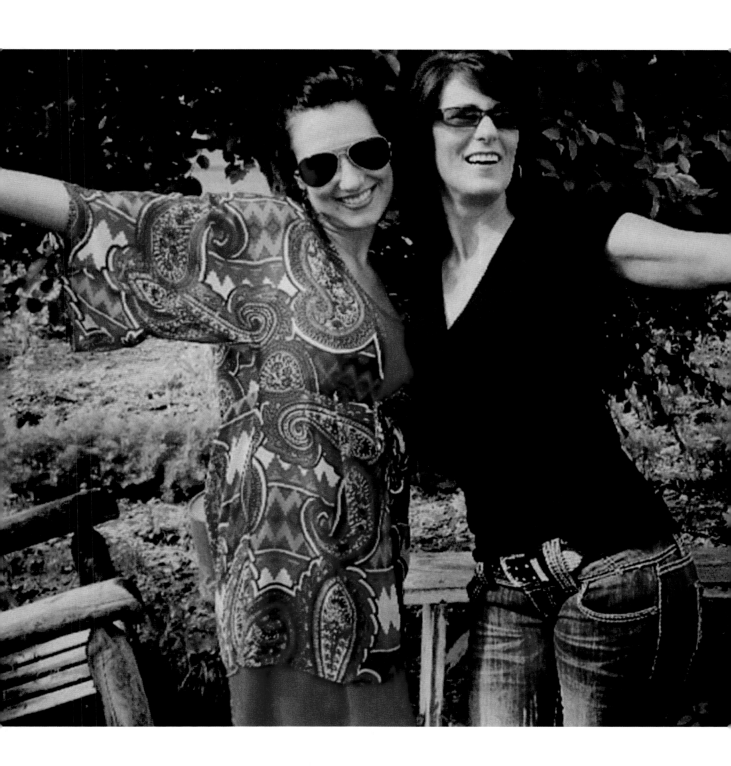

Authors
Toni Thomas & Keisha Garrett

Keisha and I wish to thank everyone who supported our efforts to bring this book to publishing and to every bride-to-be we wish you abundant joy on your wedding day!

We have confidence that you will have complete success with your DIY wedding makeup application and will look gorgeous on the most important day of your life. Using the skills we have taught you in our DIY Bridal Makeup book and putting them into practice will ultimately bring you the wedding day look you desire.

It will take time and practice but aren't you worth it?

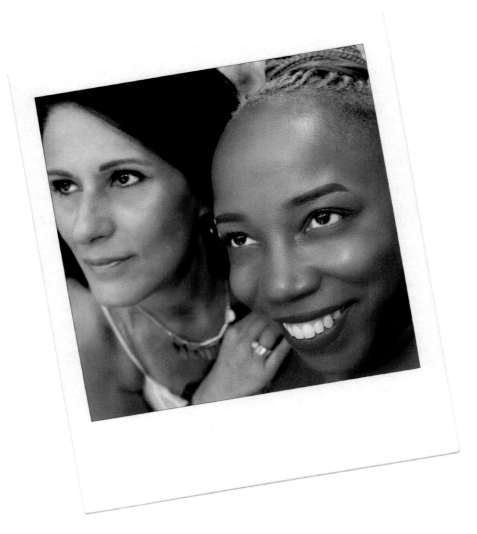

Keisha Garrett

Is a Richmond Virginia based beauty photographer and makeup artist working her passion for over twelve years, her work has been published in many magazine periodicals. She actively works her makeup and photography business everyday to bring beauty to the world through her makeup artistry and the lens of her camera. She is the mother of two gorgeous sons and one of the hardest working beauty photographers in Richmond. To be a friend of Keisha's is to have an enriched life filled with laughter, fun and joy. She follows her heart and her passions with a fierce willingness to do everything it takes to be successful.

You can find her work at keishagarret.com or KGBeautyStudio.com

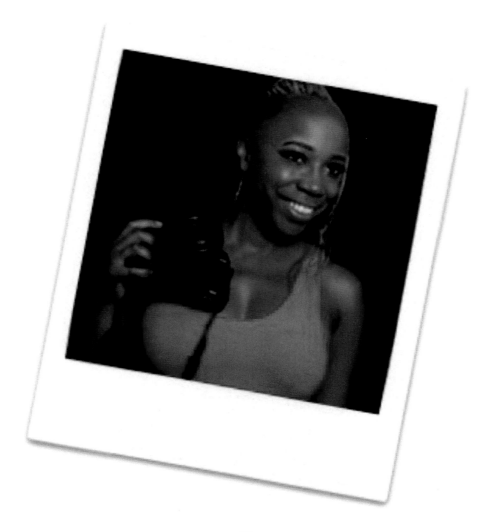

Toni Thomas

Is an Alexandria Virginia and Montana based Makeup Artist and Author, she is the founder of Women in Gear: School of Makeup Artistry, an online school that teaches makeup workshops and MUA certification classes to those who seek to enhance their makeup skills. She has been working in the beauty industry for over 23 years and has been blessed to have the opportunity to do exactly what she loves for most of her adult life. She is the mother of three beautiful children and four gorgeous grandsons. She is married to her childhood sweetheart and they are fortunate to live in beautiful Virginia as well as the mountains of Montana.

You can find her work Toni-Thomas.com or TheAmericanMakeupArtist.com you can check out her school of makeup artistry at womeningear.com.

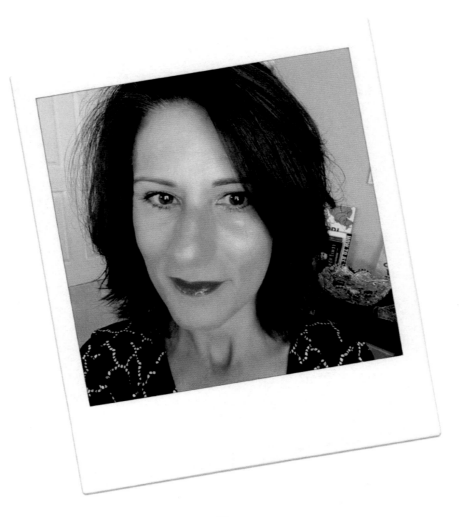

Our Brides

I have found the one whom my soul loves.

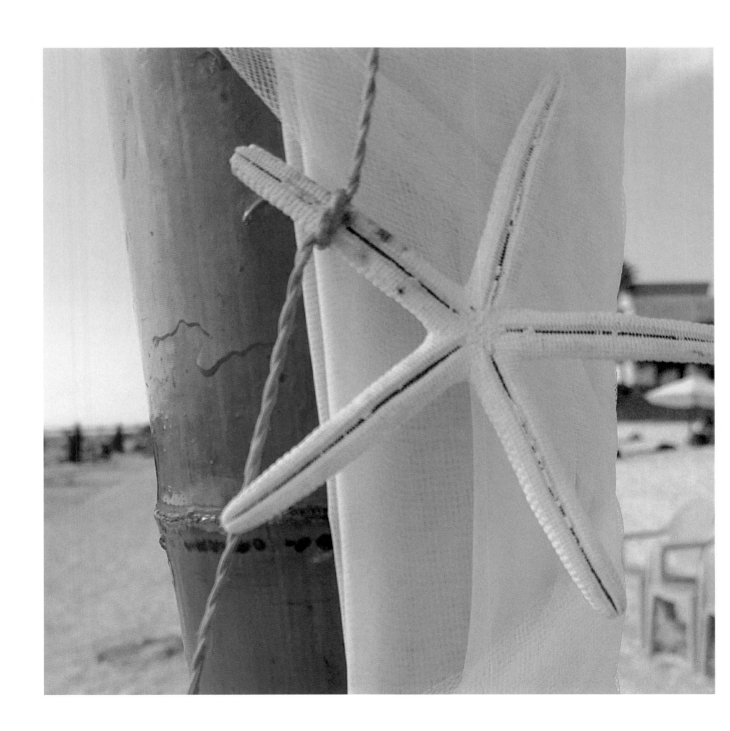

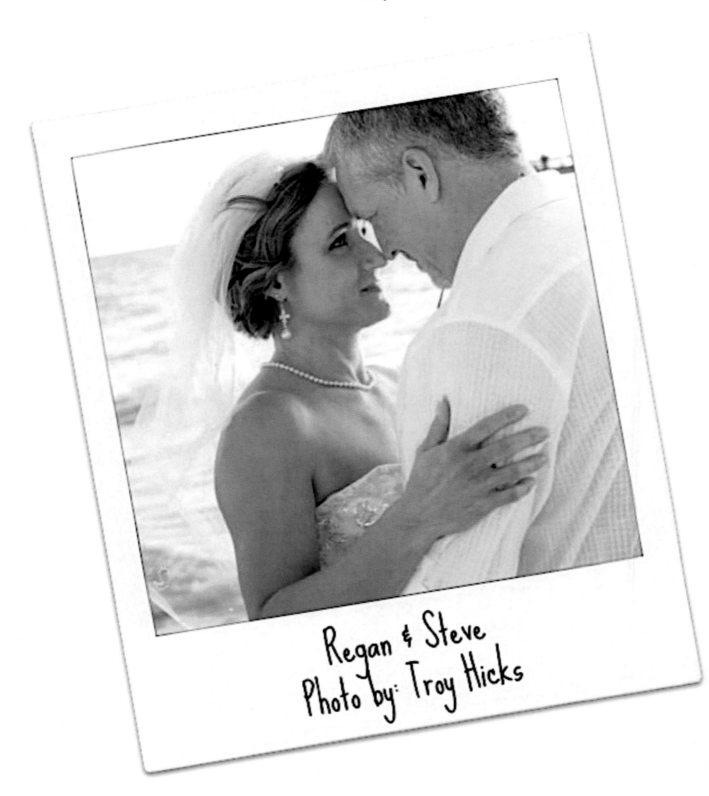

Regan & Steve
Photo by: Troy Hicks

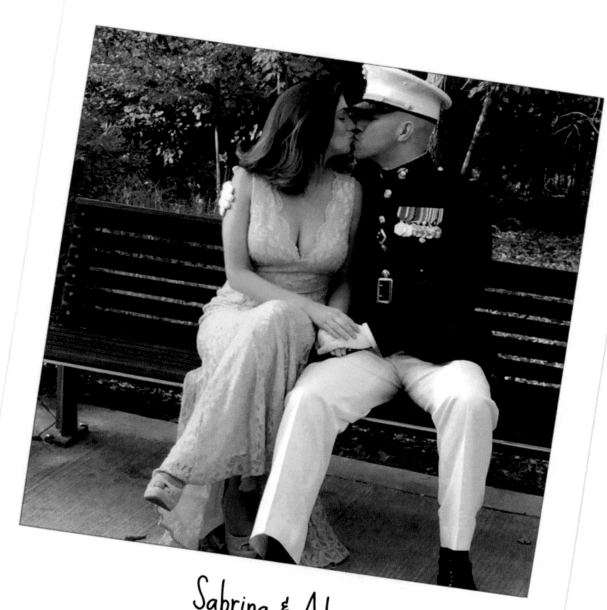

Sabrina & Adoni
Photo by: Kira Rippy

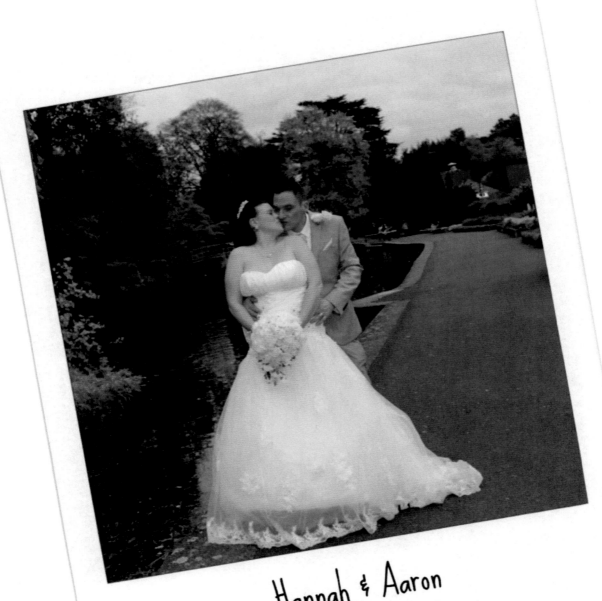

Hannah & Aaron
Photo by: Casey Anderson

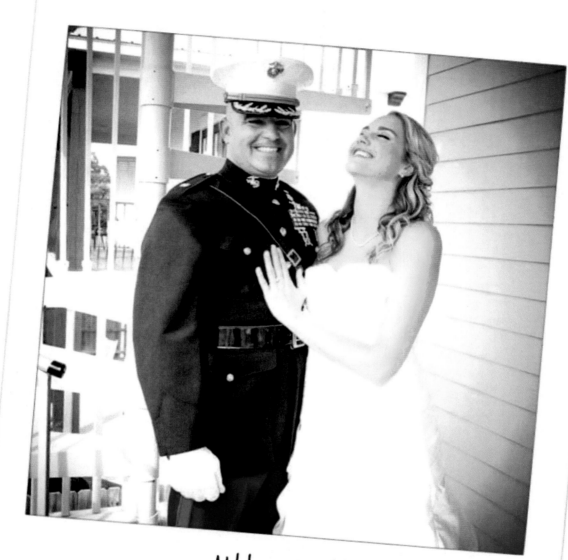

Nikki & Hank
Photo by: Angela Walsh

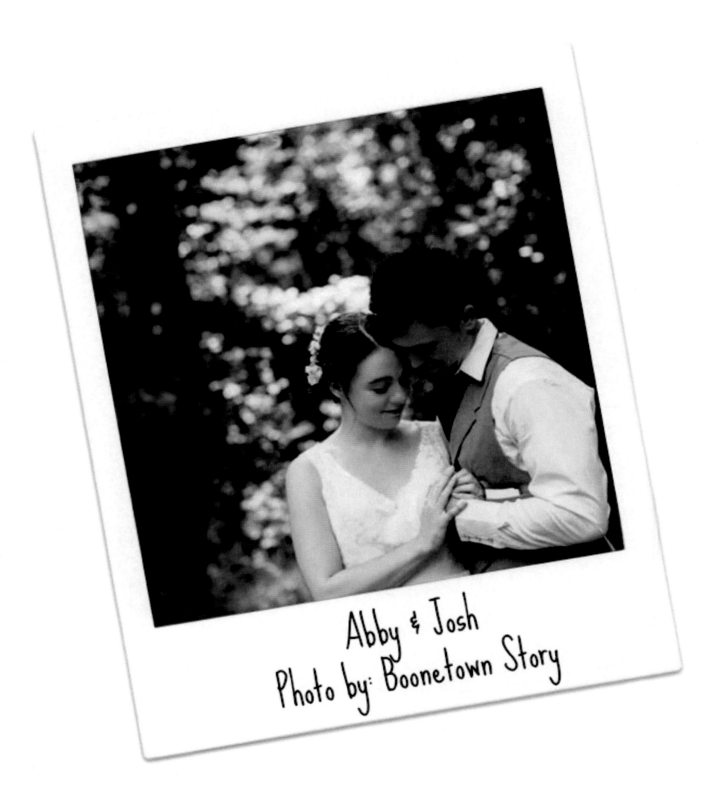

Abby & Josh
Photo by: Boonetown Story

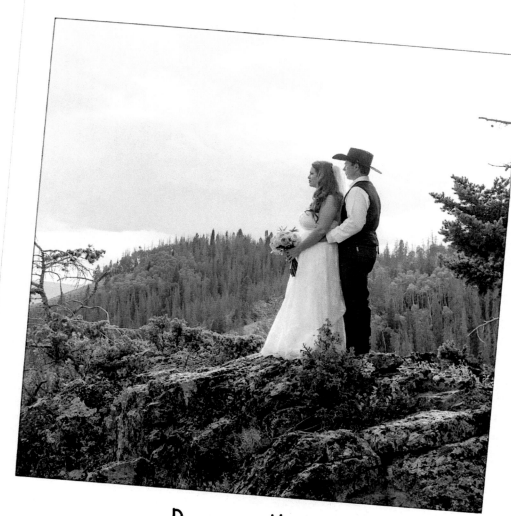

Briana & Henry
Photo by: Brian Wright

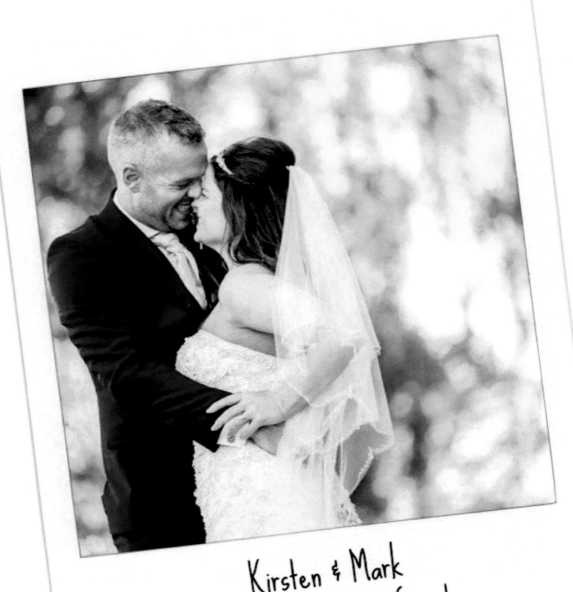

Kirsten & Mark
Photo by: Wedding Guest

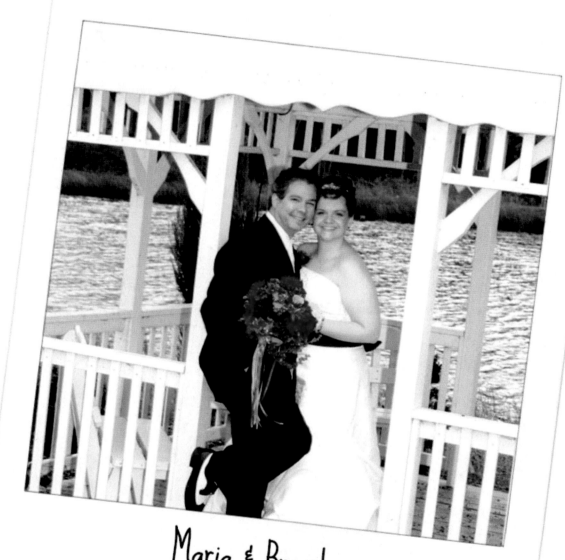

Maria & Brendan
Photo by: Jessica Bush

Bridal Extras

Bridal Hair

Doing your own hair may not be an option but if you want to attempt an easy to achieve bridal up-do we found a few easy ones to try out, all hair tutorials were found on Pinterest.

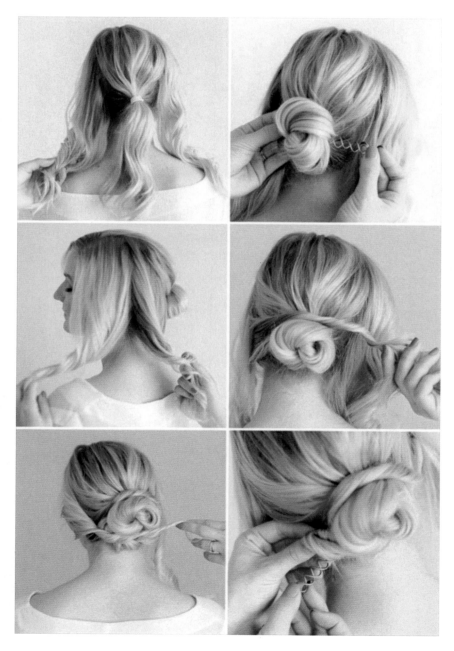

Tutorial Photos
Courtesy of Pinterest:
Source Unknown

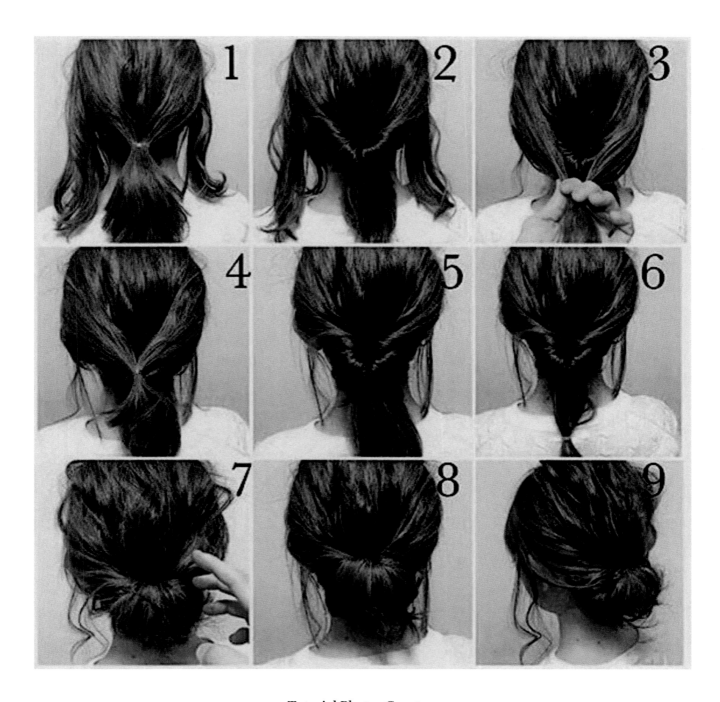

Tutorial Photos Courtesy
of Pinterest: Source
Unknown

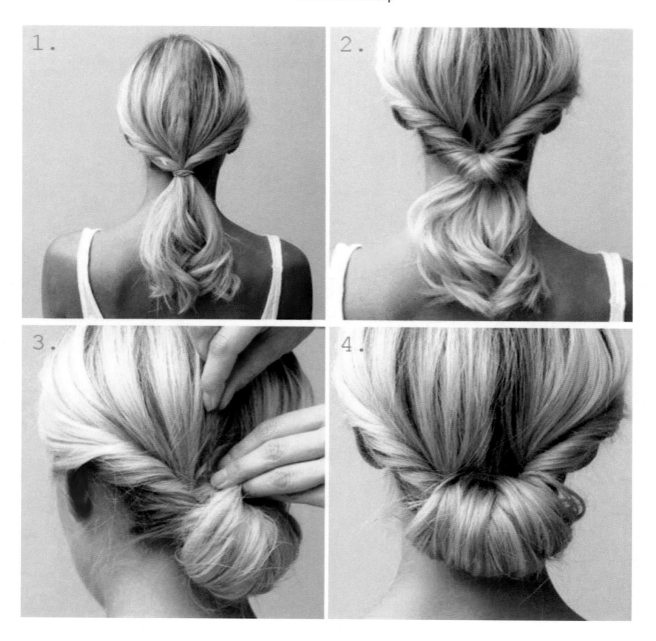

Tutorial Photos Courtesy of
Pinterest: Source Unknown

Bridal Manicure

Doing your own nails is an easy DIY option to showcase that beautiful ring on your wedding day. With a few easy strokes you can have a gorgeous manicure to highlight that beautiful new ring. We found this beautiful two-color manicure on Pinterest.

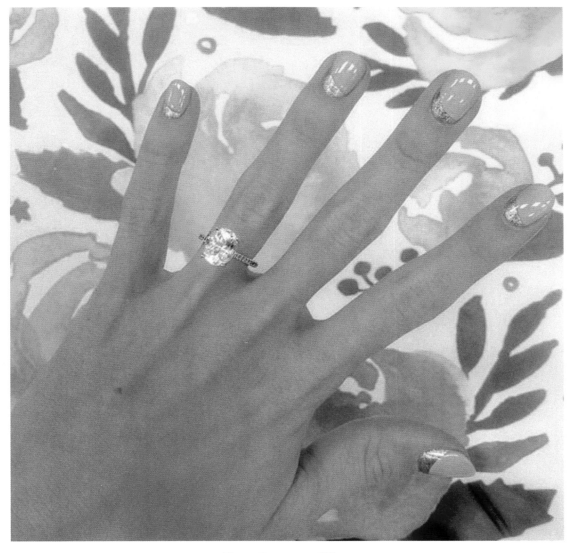

Photo Courtesy of Pinterest
Source Unknown

DIY BRIDAL MAKEUP

Your Guide to Flawless Wedding Day Makeup

Made in the USA
Las Vegas, NV
11 July 2023

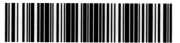